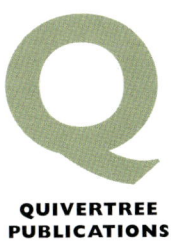

QUIVERTREE
PUBLICATIONS

WILD IRIS
herbal
HANDBOOK

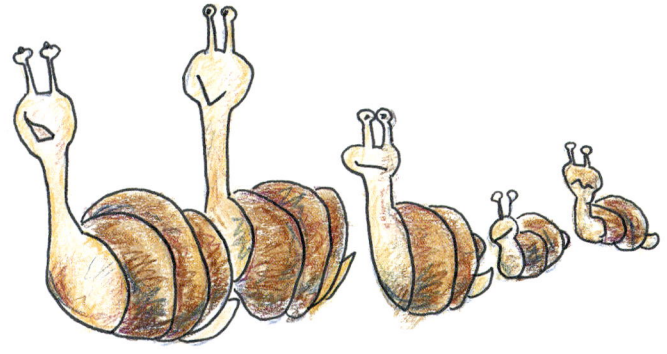

PUBLISHED BY QUIVERTREE PUBLICATIONS, SOUTH AFRICA
P O BOX 51051 • WATERFRONT • 8002 • CAPE TOWN • SOUTH AFRICA

TEL: +27 (0) 21 461 6808 • FAX: +27 (0) 21 461 6842 • E-MAIL: info@quivertree.co.za

www.quivertree.co.za

ISBN : 0-620-30667-X

ILLUSTRATIONS © SANDY MITCHELL 2003, DESIGN © QUIVERTREE PUBLICATIONS CC.® 2003.
PRINTED BY TIEN WAH PRESS, SINGAPORE. FIRST PRINTED IN 2003.
REPRODUCTION BY HIRT & CARTER CAPE (PTY) LTD

FIRST PRINTED IN 2003

THE AUTHOR IS NOT A HEALTH PRACTITIONER OF ANY KIND. ALL INFORMATION IS SOURCED AS CORRECTLY AS POSSIBLE,
BUT A HEALTH PRACTITIONER MUST BE CONSULTED FOR ALL SERIOUS AILMENTS. THE READER IS ENCOURAGED
TO SEEK ADVICE ON PLANT IDENTIFICATION IF IN DOUBT. THE PUBLISHERS AND AUTHOR CANNOT BE HELD RESPONSIBLE FOR ANY
ADVERSE REACTIONS TO HERBAL RECOMMENDATIONS OR INSTRUCTIONS. SELF-MEDICATION IS ENTIRELY AT THE READER'S OWN RISK.

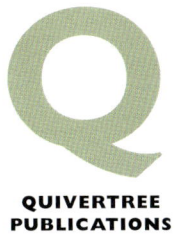

**QUIVERTREE
PUBLICATIONS**

AUTHOR: SANDY MITCHELL **| ILLUSTRATOR:** SANDY MITCHELL **| DESIGNER:** LIBBY DOYLE
PRODUCTION: LIBBY DOYLE **| SUB-EDITOR:** VERENA DOYLE

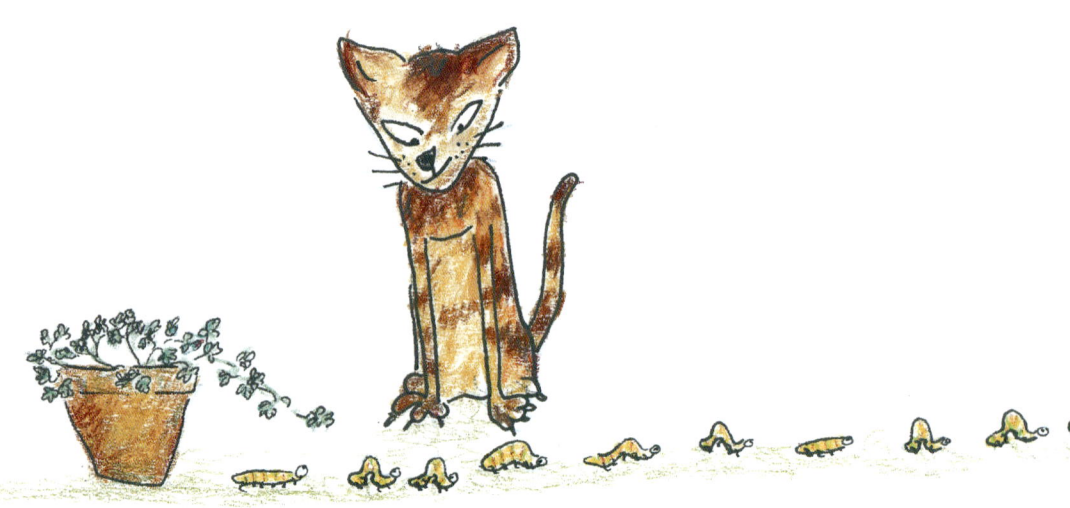

acknowledgments

Thank you for always patiently answering my embarrassingly stupid questions:
Jackie Ravenscroft - Spes Bona Herbs
Bridget Kitley, Ronald and Tony - Heiveld Herbs and Chris - Turtle Rock
(especially for making me push those laden wheelbarrows)
Libby and Craig - for laughing in all the right and wrong places,
and of course their encouragement
Hannah Hope - art critic extraordinaire

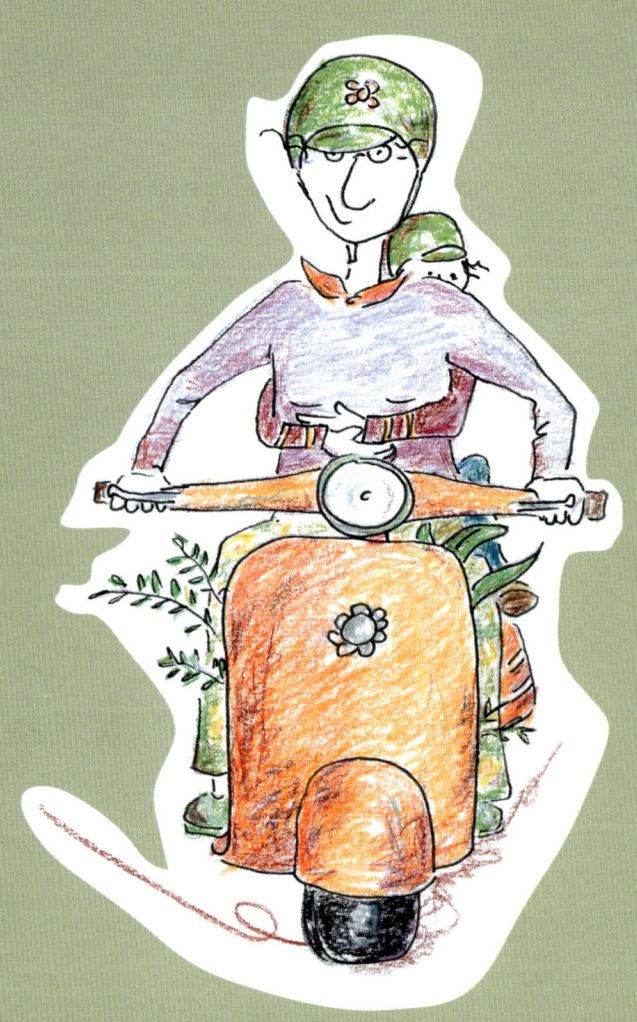

to my un-gardeners
Gabriel, Hannah, Oliver and Francis,
and of course Adrian
(meet you in the garden shed ...)

foreword

The beginnings of this book, like so many books, started as something else. When I was running my nursery I started a Newsletter, in order to lure customers to me. The idea was to inform people of the uses of herbs which would entice them to rush over and leave laden with plants, wonderfully confident with their newly acquired knowledge! The first newsletter had my husband, Adrian Hope, peering over my shoulder, saying, "It's a bit serious isn't it?". Like a sensible wife, I normally toy with throwing his advice to the wind, but I was a bit wiser this time and the result was a very popular newsletter. Gradually with the encouragement of Libby Doyle it developed into 'Wild Iris Herbal'.

I have endeavoured to follow a similar approach to the newsletter: avoiding complicated or time consuming methods in herbal preparations as most people have such busy lives, but the yearning to bring natural products into their lives and learn more about herbs is strongly there. I have also concentrated on the most readily accessible herbs as much as possible, as most have multiple uses which are so often overlooked in the search for the cure for common ailments. More complicated ailments will normally require professional assistance anyway.

I have omitted extensive details on growing herbs as I feel it is covered by so many books readily available in bookshops and libraries. More so I would like readers to be able to use this book regardless of where they live in the world.

My experience in the retail herb industry is that many people are keen to learn more about herbal usage. This book, I hope, will be an accessible introduction to herbs, as well as entice those who are already knowledgeable, and enjoy a very serious subject with a twist of humour!

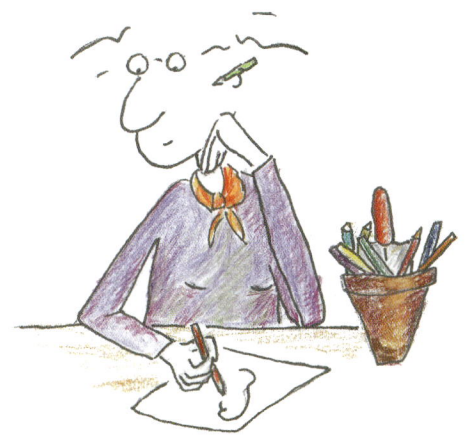

[when reading this book, if at all in doubt about proportions of herbs to use, please see pages 94-98, 'Making Herbal Preparations']

contents

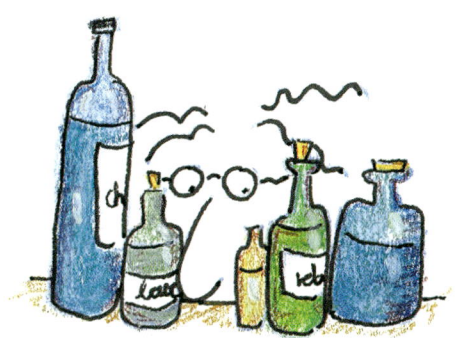

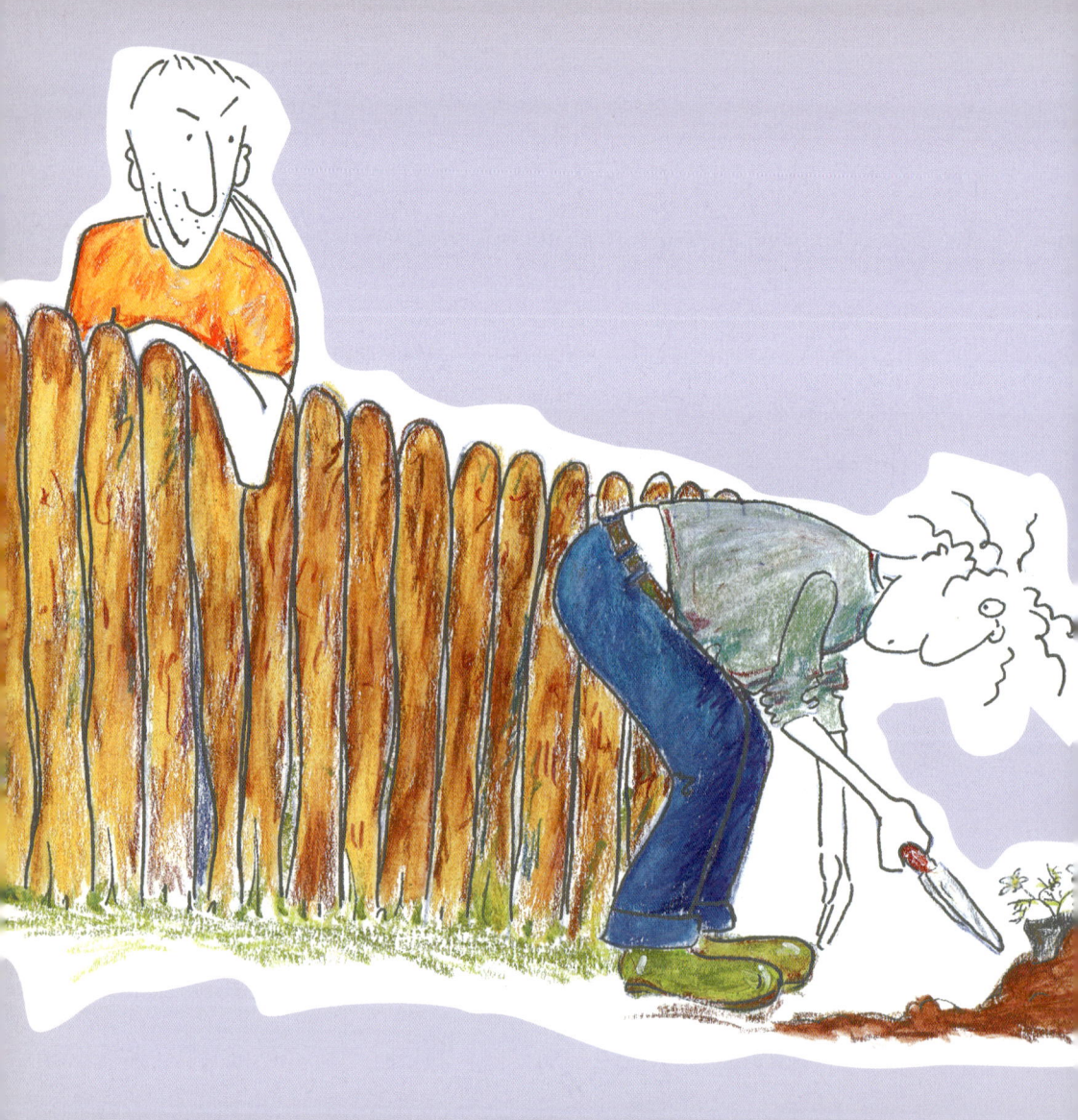

bed friends

Basil feels that Iris is his companion plant,
but Iris knows she simply, simply can't.
Hence Basil spends his days like mint,
spread over the garden fence, eyes aglint,
waiting to plant her in his garden,
feeling his soil-stained pants begin to harden.
But Iris keeps a watchful eye,
she's like a chamomile who'll die,
engulfed by such an amorous mint,
a man who never seems to get the hint,
that certain species do not grow,
side by side or in a row.
Companion plants they'll never be,
which Basil chooses not to see.

Basil & Mint

Before planting your garden or reshuffling your existing herbal cacophony into further calamity, your plants would delight in careful consideration as to who ends up with whom in the herb bed. You may find it unnecessary to have it pointed out to you that plants do not get blind drunk, wake up the next morning and find themselves in bed with a species of bad repute. However, when the garlic awakens to the whiff of peas or the parsley gets lumped with the lettuce, they cannot avoid regarding you, the gardener, as the sozzled party; wilting in each other's company. In order to successfully companion plants it would be advisable to skip the G&T and bear the role of herbal matchmaker. An exciting prospect if you consider how strawberries blush at the prospect of fruiting next to borage, or even feeling your own cheeks ripen, when dabbling in the carrot family genus feuds.

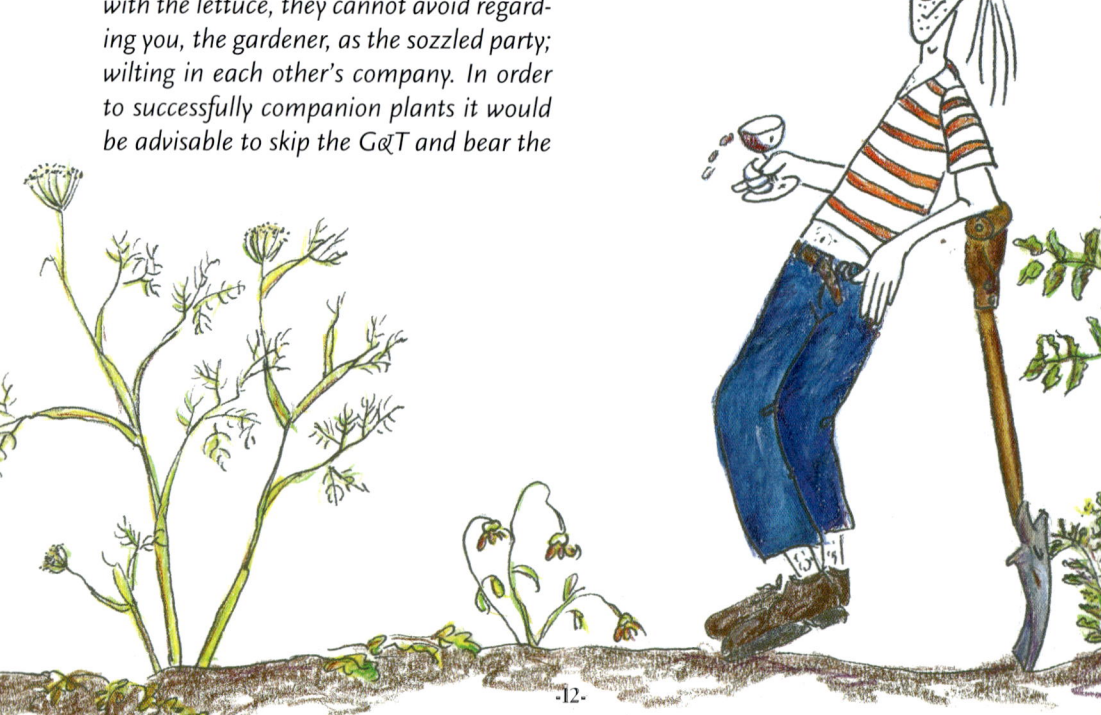

Successful garden courtship can be tricky, as we do not always know the reasons for plant preferences in choosing bed companions, but over the centuries gardeners have been able to deduce through experience that certain plants grow better in the company of particular neighbours. This is now a science labelled allelopathy. We know that chemistry plays a role in this, as well as size (naturally), compatible water needs and light. Then there is also always the good or bad body odour factor, as plants excrete substances into the air and soil, thereby making herbs oh so popular in bed. These sweet smells attract a variety of insect life, which feed off pests as well as pollinate flowers. They in turn attract other predators such as birds and so the cycle continues.

Companion plants with bad body odour can confuse insects who bypass their usual fodder, confused by the smell believed to be emitted by their usually favourite plant. Down below, root secretions help fend off disease or predators, thereby promoting strong growth.

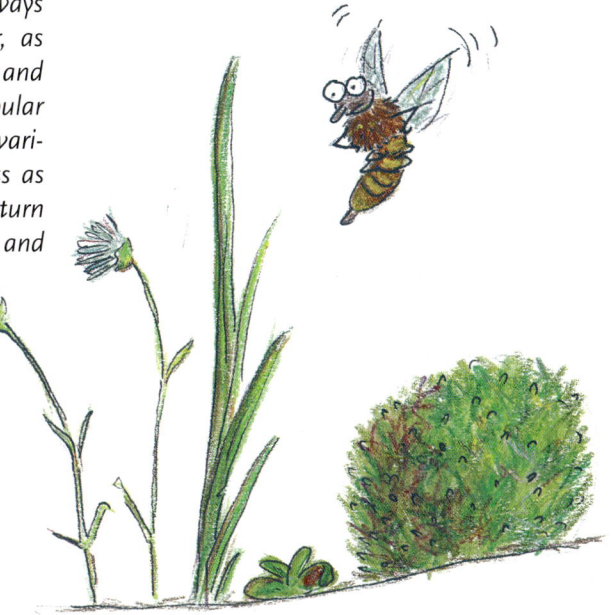

Like Jack Sprat and his wife, many plants form an agreeable marriage by eating different foods, which in turn ensure that the soil is not depleted of fertility. An assortment of root systems also breaks up the soil in varying manners, thereby releasing different organic substances and nutrients.

POPULAR BEDFELLOWS

It can be difficult to fathom the attraction of certain celebrities in the garden. Take yarrow for instance. All plants in the vicinity of this superplant fall for its flattery unerringly. Do not expect gigantic species to result from association with this fellow (size isn't everything), but rather content, healthy plants caused by yarrow's ability to increase their resistance to adverse conditions. Many plants are so enamoured of this handsome doctor, that hormones plunge into an adolescent state of titillation. The flirtatious aromatic plants are the most susceptible to yarrow's charms, resulting in super production of essential oil. And thank goodness that's all they do, as who could nurture a bed of teenage plants?

Another surprisingly popular herb is stinging nettle, the cheerleader of the garden, who stands on the side of the bed egging its fellow flora on to greater essential oil production. (All those stings are just a front.) Plants like angelica react like testosterone-filled football players, producing up to 80% more essential oil, whereas peppermint, sage and marjoram are more bashful, managing only a modest 10% increase.

Oddly, another popular type is the **marigold (tagetes sp.).** *These ugly ducklings manage to turn tomatoes and potatoes into swans,* but are so foul smelling that even the nasty nematodes pack their bags for the neighbour's garden, making it every plant's desire to snuggle up to this Mexican wonder. White flies too join the exodus from marigolds, leaving carrots much relieved, and the gardener confused as to how to plant this beneficial plant everywhere, without its being smelt.

As herbal matchmaker, you will find it useful to know that carrots love chives and onion, whereas sweet smelling roses are attracted to sulphuric garlic. Parsley will sidle up to roses as well as to tomatoes. Rosemary, the hussy, will leap into bed with sage at any given opportunity. But please bear in mind that there can also be some seriously ...

Carrots, chives + onions
Roses + garlic + sage

● BAD MATCHMAKING

In love some plants (and people) can be blissfully blind. Watch how peppermint oozes with oil next to chamomile, who in turn cringes with horror at the touch of this gushing mint. If you love chamomile, please spare it this embarrassment. On the whole, the mint family is in ill-repute as bedhogs.

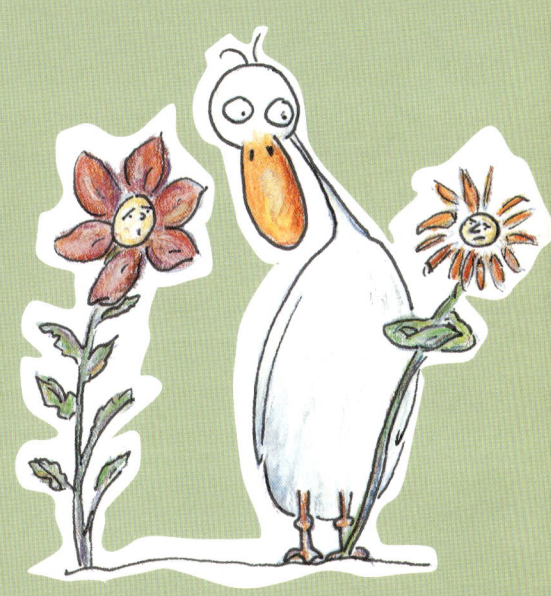

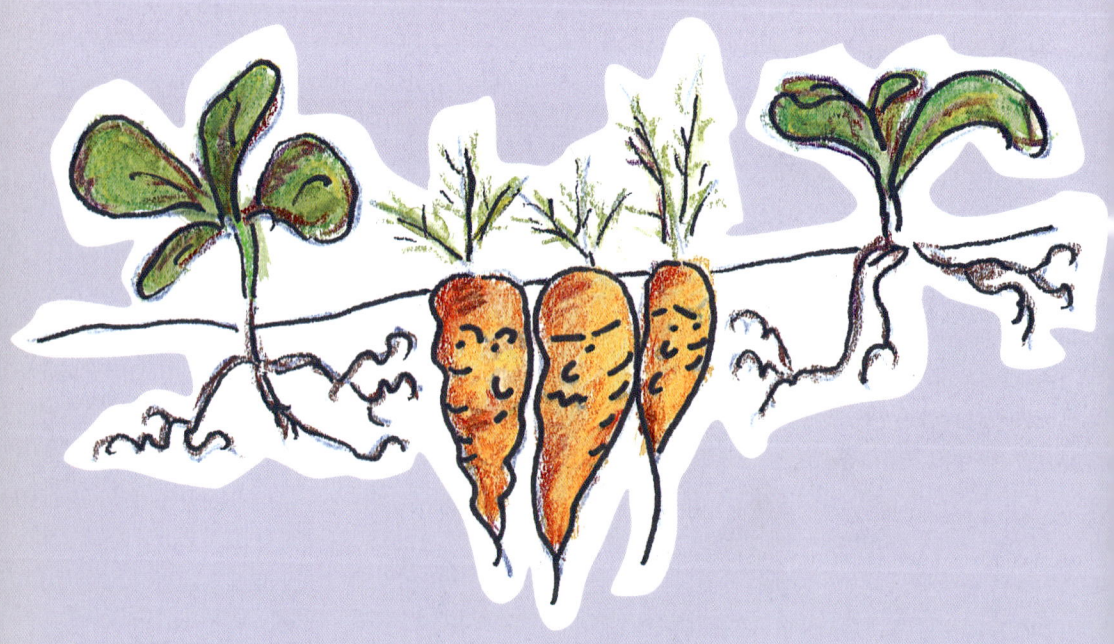

How can any decent upright plant grow when enmeshed by the amorous affections of creepy menthe? Don't abandon this over zealous herb though, just give it its own bed and yank it out at the merest sign of it attempting to sidle up to the prissy parsley. Mint does keep your breath fresh and the insects repelled, so it is worth planting. (Separate bedrooms though!)

Uncomfortable family dynamics can also creep into your soil. Herbs like fennel should not share a bed with its relatives. (Most sensible!) This seedy character is prone to bad relations with its cousins dill, coriander, caraway and chervil and even certain vegetables, like beans and tomatoes, will clarify that fennel has a grumpy disposition and will not grow near it. Wormwood, however, has the upper hand over fennel, creating such panic it hinders germination. Talking of wormwood, some plants would rather die than share their beds with a plant with such infamous body odour. Have a cup of wormwood tea and you'll find yourself partial to this opinion. Fortunately, it is not only plants that find this herb distasteful, but also pests, caterpillars in particular. So plant it near for pest control, but at a safe distance.

Further bad bedmate decisions include dandelion, who is often black mouthed by other plants. It cannot help exhaling ethylene gas, but other foliage simply won't grow with that in their transpiration passages. So zap it and brew it; your compost will be delighted.

Don't be deceived by the sweet façade of certain aromatics such as lavender. It can be quite the bed hog, to the detriment of the other charmers nearby. Other incompatible relationships include rue and basil. Keep your basil with tomatoes and rue should stick to roses and raspberries. That is if you wish to remain running for nomination of 'gardener of the year' by your protégés.

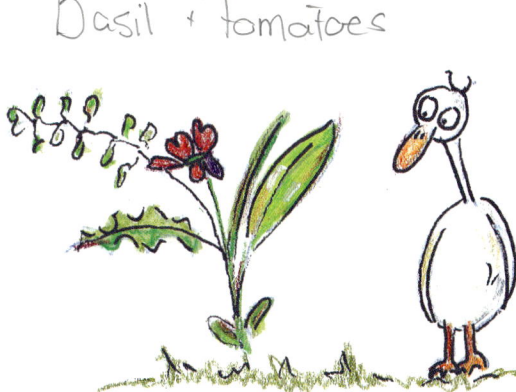

Basil + tomatoes

Remember that the position of garden matchmaker requires a roving eye to nourish good relationships as well as facilitate a few divorces. Use the tried and tested combinations, but also experiment with other herbs and scented plants, especially those found in your local region.

Happy bed hopping ...

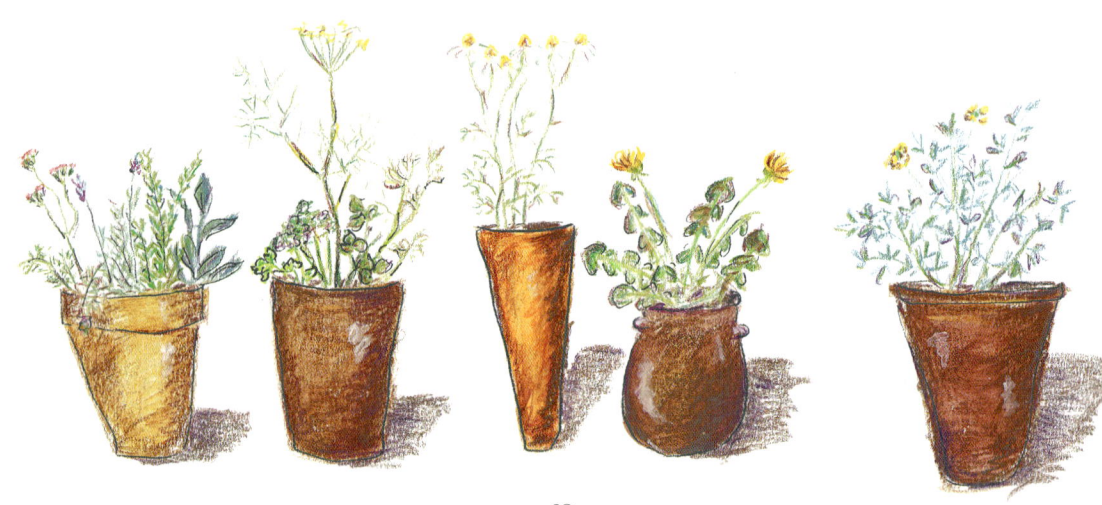

	basil	fennel	borate	dill	caraway	sage	wormwood	rosemary	mint	chamomile	chives	chervil	garlic	hyssop	nasturtium	parsley	savoury	thyme
tomatoes	✔	✗							✗							✔		
beans	✔	✗									✗		✗				✔	
rue	✗																	
strawberries			✔													✔		
cabbage			✔	✔	✔	✔	✔	✔	✔				✗			✔		✔
onions				✔								✔					✔	
carrots				✗		✔		✔		✔	✔							
radishes												✔		✗	✗			
corn				✔														
lettuce				✔												✗		
cucumber				✔									✔					
caraway		✗																
dill		✗																
coriander		✗																
wormwood		✗																
peas													✗					
potatoes							✔								✗			
sage		✗																
roses						✔							✔					
beetroot													✔					

oddballs

Life has got its oddballs, it's plain enough to see,
But have you ever thought, if that applies to me;
Like Iris in her office, sorting out long data,
when her head is in the garden, singing a sonata.
The indoor life is stifling, her colleagues think her odd,
she smiles benignly, the polite society nod.

Computer screens have colour, but lack in floral scent,

Iris knows not why the hours are not rather spent,

Brewing up concoctions, to nurse an ailing plant,

or cutting back verbena, to a Tibetan Buddhist chant.

But gardening is not all relaxation,
or twentieth century meditation,
It's sweat, slog and labour, but passion at its best,
sorting out the oddballs from the rest.
But it doesn't buy her butter, it doesn't buy her bread,
so she tackles keyboards and monitors instead

At work, others indulge in lunchtime pixel smut,
But Iris is no computer worldwide slut,
instead, her hand deflowers the garden herbal sites,
(all gardeners are endowed with certain given rights)
whilst other drool at human flesh seduction,
Iris slobbers at floral reproduction.

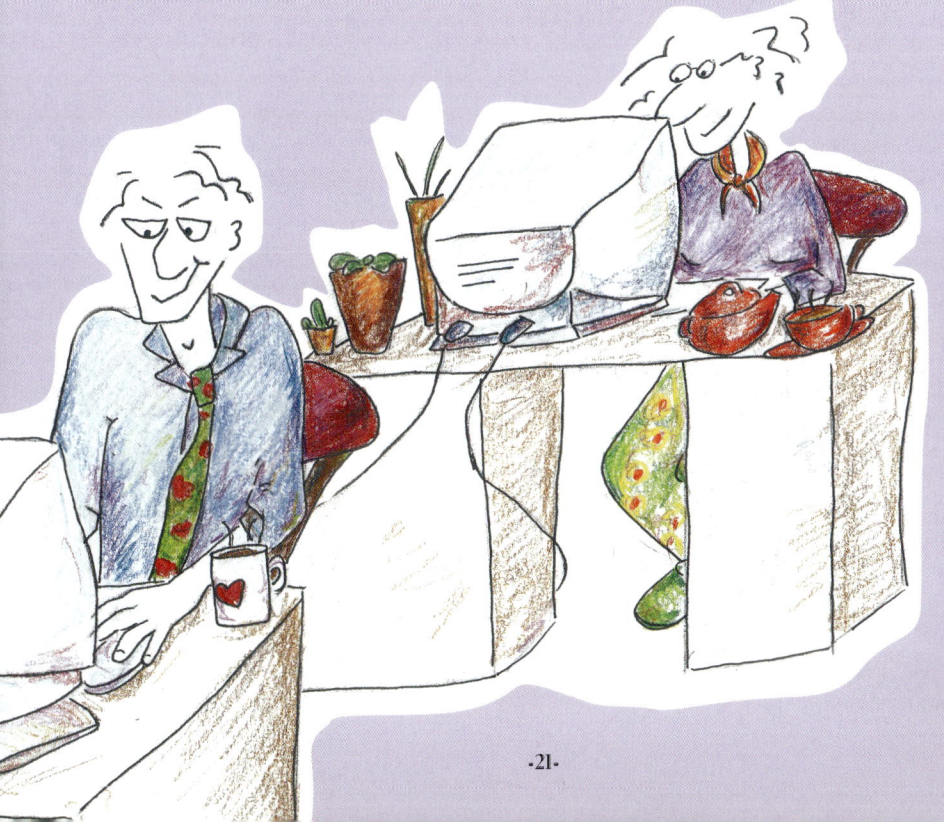

Any amount of time spent 'people watching' will remind us of the truism that some of us are odder than others. The same can be said of plants and thus we often neglect the strange, non-conformist plants, by sticking to the conventional, humming, 'parsley, sage, rosemary and thyme', as we plow the garden bed. Be reminded though, that a herb is merely a useful plant, so change your ditty to 'alfalfa, artichokes and senna'.

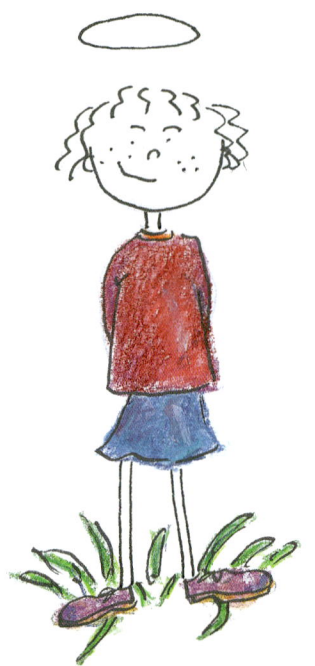

Angelica (Angelica archangelica)

There are few herbs that will grow in the shade and that is why Angelica is the darling of shady herb gardens. It is also tall growing (up to two metres) and therefore makes a good backdrop; besides, it is difficult to resist cultivating a plant baptised Angelica archangelica. This herb showers us with its blessing in the form of biennial seeds which germinate in and around the garden with gay abandon. Do take note though, that they are not of the earthly kind and cannot be stored, as they will lose viability. Choose deep, rich, moist and slightly acidic soil for Angelica with a bit of morning sun. You can prolong its life on earth by decapitating its seed head in the second year, enabling it to persevere a year or two longer.

Cook Angelica leaves and stems with stewed fruit, as well as when making jams, to neutralise their acidity. Young stems can be added raw to salad and children enjoy chewing them, which has the added benefit of easing carsickness. Angelica is known to stimulate circulation and digestion as well as cleanse the liver. It has a calming effect on the digestive tract, eliminates flatulence as well as eases colic pains. This guardian angel also strengthens the lungs by working as a tonic. It is also useful for cystitis and menstrual irregularities and pain.

Cayenne (Capsicum frutescens)

All gardens should be bedecked with chillis, but cayenne in particular has its place in the medicinal herb garden. The traffic light colours of these plants certainly stop the eye from roaming, and its taste is bound to bring you to a screeching halt, but wait, there's more to cayenne than the spice kitchen will tell. Not surprisingly improved circulation is hot on the cards, as well as cayenne's toning and strengthening effect on the heart and blood vessels. Believe it or not, this firecracker has a toning effect on the digestive system as it improves digestion and eases flatulence. Naturally, it promotes perspiration and warms a feverish system, but do not use medicinally if pregnant, breastfeeding or suffering from gastric ulcers.

Alfalfa/Lucerne (Medigo sativa)

Join old MacDonald and his herd by introducing this herb to your garden. Use the leaves, young shoots and sprouts in salads. The benefits are unbearably good. Seeds are best sought out at a health shop but sometimes supermarkets will endow you with it.

Why chew the cud? Well if it's good enough for prize-winning Arab horses, it's good enough for your salad bowl. Just say 'neigh' and get on with it, as you will be consuming every vitamin you require in the process (beat that), as well as a good cudful of minerals. It helps reduce uric acid and relieves some forms of arthritis, gout and rheumatism. Convalescents will find it helpful as an appetite stimulant. Now where would you find a vitamin pill that produces attractive violet flowers as well as so much chlorophyll? Plant it in rich soil and allow it to bask in the sun. Allow some seeds to multiply effortlessly in your garden.

Stinging Nettle (Urtica urens/dioca)

Many of you will balk at the idea of cultivating this terrorist of all weeds, particularly if most of your weekends are spent employing guerrilla garden techniques to eradicate it. Back off and befriend nettle as it has excellent medicinal properties. The young leaves are selected, as the raw older ones can cause kidney damage. If you don't already have the pleasure of nettle invasion in your garden it can be grown in semi-shade in dampish soil, best in a large container. When it gets out of hand, punish it with the compost heap, as it is an excellent activator.

What does this notorious weed have for you? It will rid your body of excess uric acid and has a cleansing effect on kidneys. Externally nettle tincture or lotion is soothing and healing for both eczema and urticaria. Nettle is both cleansing and a tonic, rich in minerals, especially Vitamin C and iron. It is therefore good and safe for pregnant women, or anaemics. When nursing, nettle will give you the vitamins required as well as improve milk supply. Young nettle leaves can also be used to make a delicious soup.

Chaste Tree (Vitex agnes castus)

Chastity is not quite the word to describe the modern lifestyle, but for men wishing to decrease their sexual desire this is the tree for you. (Any takers?) The opposite is true for women, and especially if you suffer from hormonal irregularities, particularly menopausal women. Chaste tree will balance errant hormones.

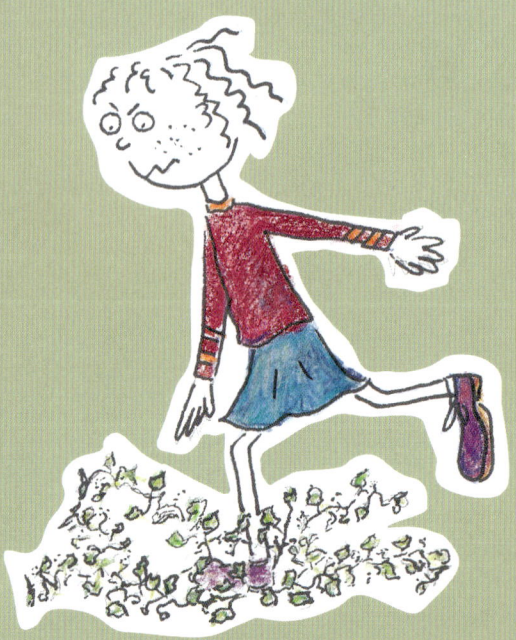

If you wish to sneak this herb into your partner's aperitif for either reason, use the dried fruit. If your hormones behave in general, then enjoy the attractive lilac panicles of flowers. It grows about six metres high and is deciduous.

Horseradish (*Armorica rusticana*)

Not quite an oddball, but most people are nervous of planting horseradish, perhaps because it is dedicated to a lifetime's relationship with you and your garden, often sneaking up on your other plants in the least expected places, but it can be put to good use and you don't even have to sacrifice a cow to enjoy it as a condiment. Before we get to the dinner banquet, horseradish is happiest in a light, well-composted soil with sun. It may take up to two to three years to get the long roots you require in autumn. They should obviously be washed and then grated or sliced. To preserve, immerse the whole root in vinegar. Next, your dinner plate - add to sauces and vinegars. Grate into coleslaw, dips, pickled beetroot, mayonnaise and avocado dips.

The fresh root contains calcium, magnesium, Vitamin C and a natural antibiotic.

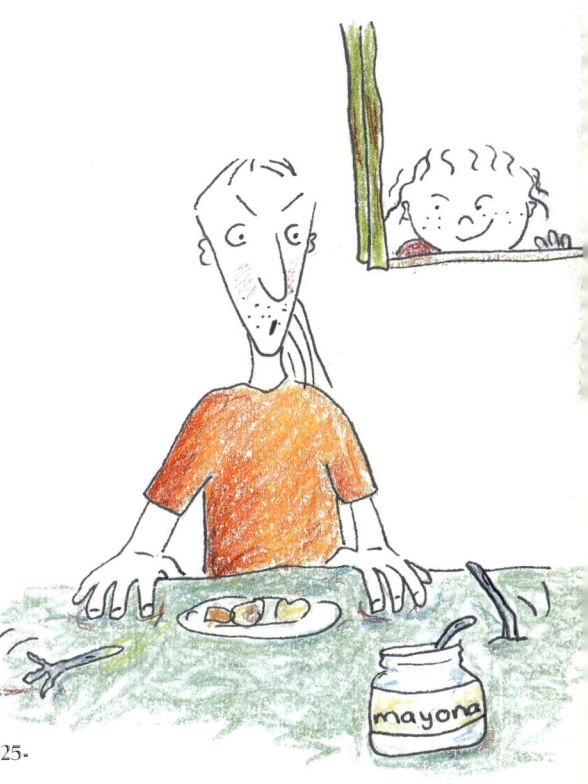

Artichoke (Cynara scolymus)

No oddball could be more pleasing than an artichoke, or more delightful, an entire row of them. If your aesthetic eyeball has never been initiated by an artichoke flower, then consider yourself trapped in the floral dark ages. 'Luminous' is the word to best describe this purple bloom and when it goes to seed it shoots out rockets of progeny to parachute down into the beckoning earth.

With artichokes comes the greatest decision in plant/stomach history. To eat or to bloom, as it is the bud of this royal coloured flower that we allow butter to slide down, before appeasing our taste buds. The answer would lie in abundance, allowing the surplus to stage their beauty pageant.

Senna (Senna alexandrina)

Don't try and fool me that you don't get the occasional blocked sewerage canal and have to call in the plumber. There are herbs for the gasworks and there are also herbs to get the show on the road. A member of the legume family, this plumber is daintier than the average

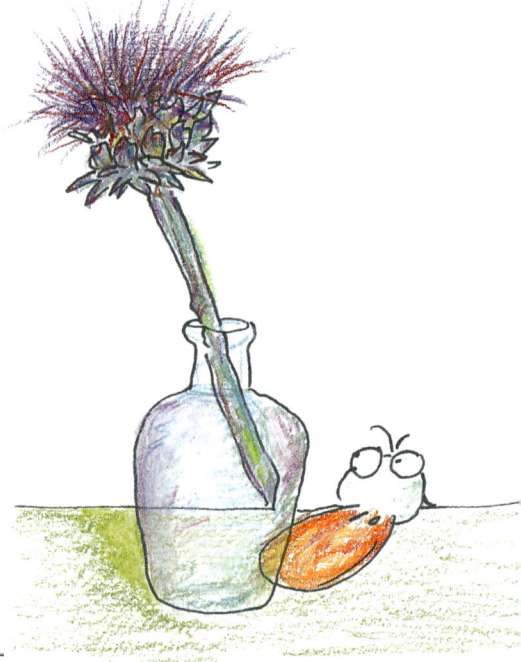

handyman with pretty yellow pea-like flowers. It is the pods that are used so you do not have to sacrifice its floral bits to your dark internal chasm. Once dried, they can be stored in an airtight container for a lengthy period or you can increase your supply by sowing the seeds. Like any good tradesman this herb will cleanse the unseen parts and stimulate them into working order. They should also cause an evacuation of worms. Grow in well-drained soil in full sun. It has the tendency to be withdrawn in winter but resumes its normal spark in spring.

Borage (Borago officinalis)

Although found in many herb gardens, borage deserves the oddball award for its remarkable interior qualities in the face of a suspicious exterior. It's not that the cornflower blue starry flowers are not aesthetically arresting, but it fails to meet the standards laid out by many other herbs for feel good, smell good qualities, through its hairy leaves and insipid aroma. However, borage's prickly skin well conceals its potassium and calcium rich exterior, which is worthwhile including in a salt free diet. Furthermore an infusion of these seemingly inhospitable leaves acts as a tonic, especially useful as an adrenal gland stimulant. Because of this action an infusion of leaves is valuable after a period of stress or depression, as well as following cortisone or steroid treatment. As a febrifuge, borage can also be taken with feverish colds and flu.

The attractive flowers are added to drinks and fruit salad, but are really best shown off adorning a chocolate cake! When the flowers are permitted to go to seed, an extraction of starflower oil containing Gamma Lineolic Acid is made or can be bought. This is recommended for menstrual problems, blood pressure, arthritis and irritable bowels.

Believe it or not, borage can be added to your dinner, finely chopped into cream cheese or yoghurt; the bristly hairs will go undetected. Those fearful of a hairy tongue may cook them with spinach, ravioli, cucumber soup or cabbage for its mild cucumber flavour.

the good, the bad and the crunchy

Could it really be nutritious,
what Angelica finds delicious?
As Iris pleads to watch a leaf go past,
the lips declaring a chlorophyll-free fast,
as underneath the table, it is not a dog that waits,
but rather a host of snails, fattened by the salads on her plate.

"Give me ice cream and chocolate cake,
white bread with smudgeons of butter,
for goodness sake,
perhaps some olive oil on pasta,
anything greasy is on my roster,
but don't catch me putting leaves upon my plate.
For that you'll simply have to wait,
until you've managed to hybridise
a milkshake flavoured lettuce leaf surprise"

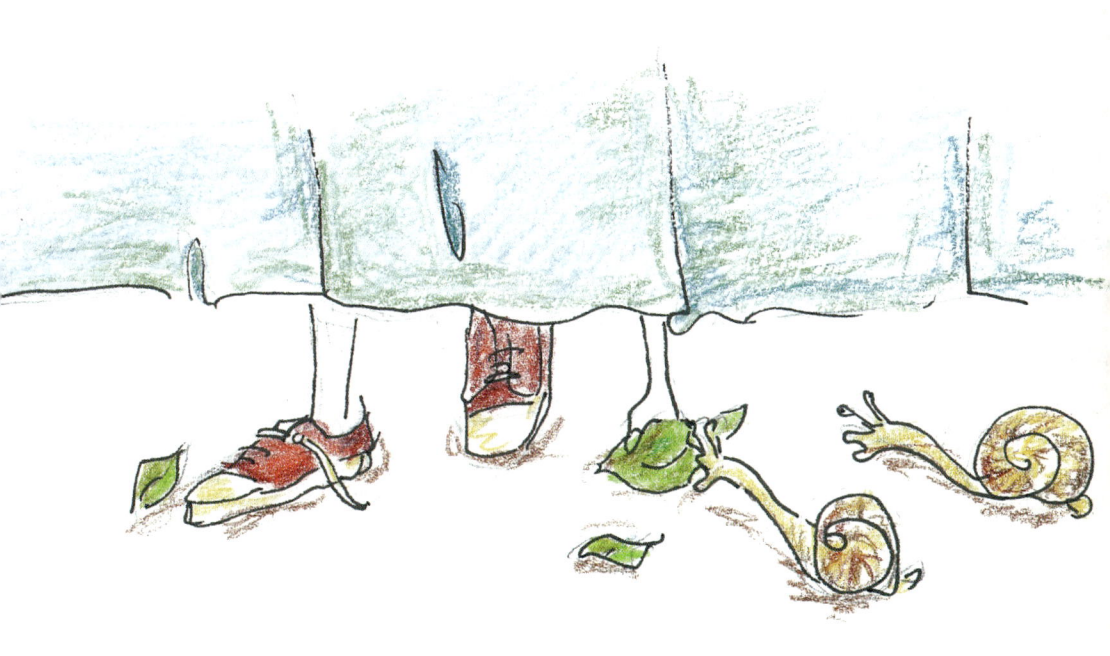

Nature presents a lot of soppy stuff we get to ooh and aah about, but certain creatures debilitate the aesthetic eye more than others. *In fact the quicker we dispose of, say, slugs, the quicker our eye can roam onto the burgeoning pink blossoms.* The problem is that being dirty fingered gardeners who need to hang on to a few romantic tenets about nature, we are compelled to find something admirable about mobile mucous. After all, such relentless consumption of greenery can't come easy. Why do slugs spend their short lifespan chomping salad and other edible greens?

The answer may lie in the green captivation of the light of the sun, or more blandly known as chlorophyll, that we pile onto our plates and buff up with olive oil and balsamic vinegar. Yes, green, nature's finest healer, high in oxygen, beneficial to all body and brain tissues and a well-trained bodyguard against intruder bacteria. Chlorophyll is also known to neutralise toxins in our bodies and anaemia sufferers should follow the beaten slug path, to boost their haemoglobin production.

A little discernment is useful when preparing the salad bowl, as there is lettuce and there is, well, lettuce. There are however also tasty and healthy green herbs, which remain unbashful of the salad dressing. Just pick out the slugs ...

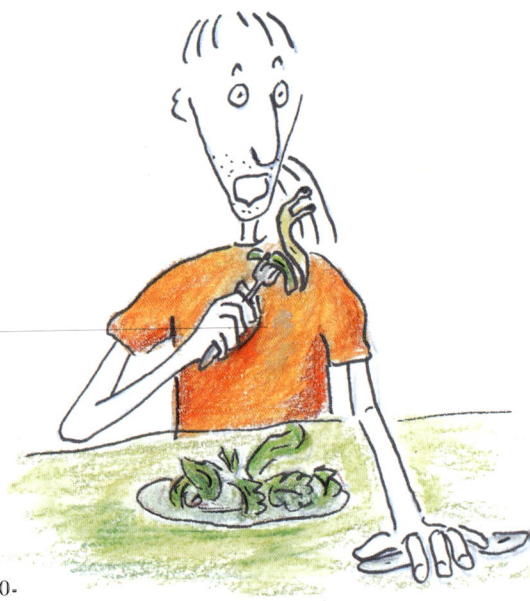

THE LETTUCE SHY SALAD ...

Reserve your judgment of gastropods and follow the gluey path of your garden foe. Devoid of salad bowl, this pest tosses its greens inwards, leaving a luminous green trail for you to fume at. With scant hesitation it sloths its way towards the chives. Whether you throw this into stews, soups or rice dishes, the slug cares not. It is a salad eater and the mild onion flavour cannot be passed.

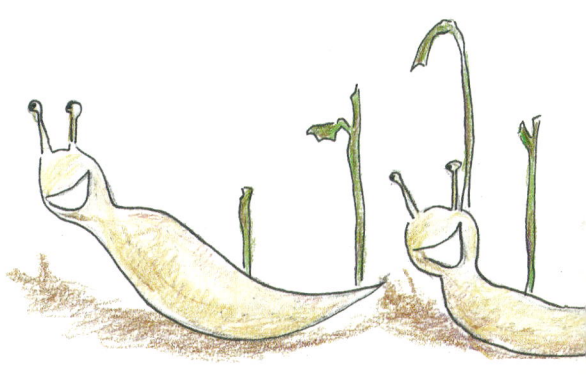

*Next on the slug hors d'oeuvre map is parsley to cleanse its breath of onion, but also ensuring it gets its Vitamin C and iron helpings. Restrain yourself from mezze luna-ing the **parsley (Petroselinum sp.)** (especially as you might not have noticed the slug), rather break small pieces into the salad.*

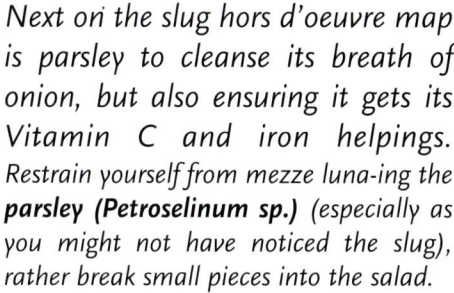

This renowned herb is more than just a pretty sprig tossed onto the side of your plate. Polite dinner guests, requiring breath freshening, will appreciate the opportunity to chomp it after your serving of roast chicken with whole head of garlic, and at the same time benefit from

improved digestion. A most subtle way to offer this service would be to find it in a salad, or on the other hand it would be delighted to find itself in soup, omelettes, rice dishes and toasted sandwiches. As it is a diuretic, arthritis suffers should eat it on a daily basis. The tastiest parsley, according to both slugs and my taste buds, is the flat/Italian leaved version (Petrosileum crispum var. neopolitanum), which is also the hardier version to grow. Be reminded though that folklore holds that only a witch or pregnant women can successfully grow this herb, so if you're not pregnant, keep your successful parsley propagation hushed.

Continue the slug meander towards the explosive taste of **rocket (Eruca vesicaria ssp. sativa).** This has nothing to do with astral travel or space suits, merely a whimsical Anglicisation of the French 'rocquette'. It is a nutty, mustardy herb with great cleansing qualities (ask your slugs) as well as having the ability to fix vitamin deficiencies and digestive upsets. **When it is not orbiting in your salad bowl, you should try it with fish, aubergine, tomatoes or green beans.** Add it to warm dishes at the end of cooking.

Heading more towards the slug meal of the day is the pleasantly leafy leaf, **chicory (Cichorium intybus)**. Your association with this herb may have more to do with brown granules posing as coffee. (Which slugs know nothing about of course.) These are the ground roots, which are often added to instant coffee, whereas the blanched leaf can be eaten raw or cooked. **Advantages of this as a salad plant are that it eliminates uric acid from the body and assists haemoglobin in its fight against anaemia**. If this plant never enters your mouth, at least your eyes will be seduced by its attractive cornflower blue spring blooms. (That is if the slugs leave you any.)

Mustardy herbs, like **nasturtium (Tropaelum majus)**, add that extra bite to your salad, even when not nursing a sore throat or cold, **with its antibiotic qualities.** Slugs of course find these medicinal qualities superfluous, but love its strong mustard leaves. These (the leaves, not the slugs) taste delicious in rice dishes and in soups. If you require a gentler taste, there is the wonderfully perennial **salad burnett (Sanguisorba minor),** which exudes a mild cucumber taste. Bear in mind that the Romans used this to staunch wounds, so it could come in handy when attacked by the mezze luna!

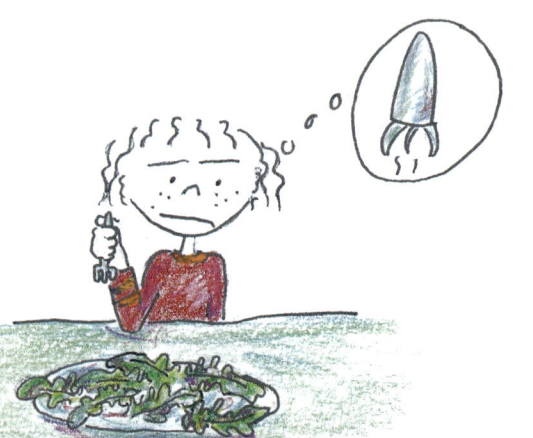

You may be surprised to find that slugs enjoy fresh young **lovage (Levisticum officinale)** leaves for their digestive and flatulence easing properties. For humans it is also useful as a blood cleanser as well as increasing haemoglobin. The taste is similar to celery with a slight licorice flavour. Stay away from older leaves which become bitter (and twisted), leaving them for the more sluggish of salad eaters. Follow the medieval practice of placing lovage in your shoes to counteract smelly and **weary feet**, but not very edible following this treatment!

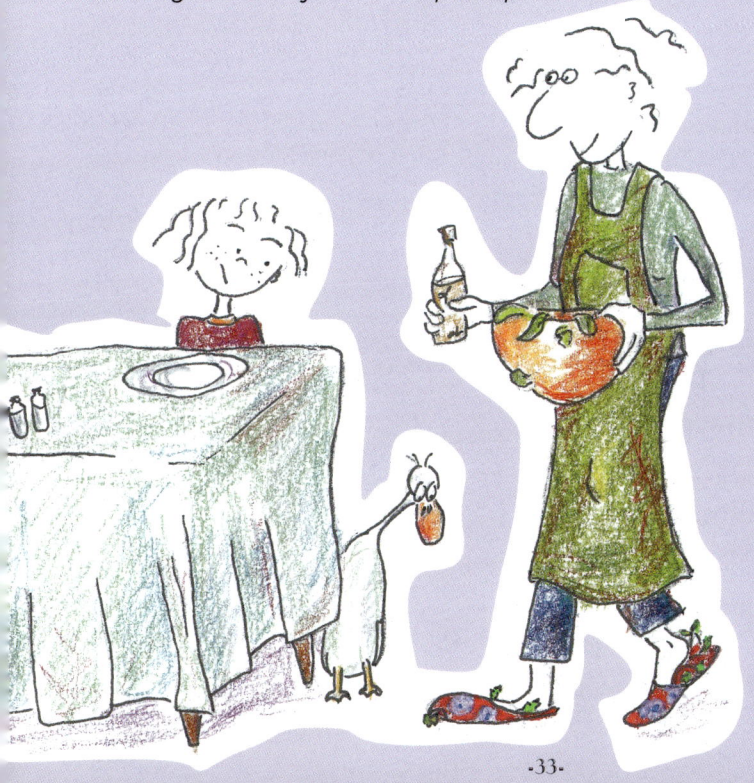

Cousins **fennel (Foeniculum vulgare)** and **chervil (Anthriscus cerefolium)** all taste best before their umbrella of seeds unfolds. The Lenten herb, chervil is rich in Vitamin C, iron and magnesium, and cleanses the blood. As a digestive and circulation stimulant it makes an excellent sweet tasting winter herb.

When it comes to serving dinners, which have your guests struggling to stifle their bottoms from rumbling in on the conversation, make sure you've added some fennel to the salad. When not counteracting flatulence or colic, this herb is good for liver regeneration. The licorice taste of fennel makes it well crunched by children in the garden and not too badly munched by slugs, who find all that extraneous information useless.

Before you toss in the **coriander (Coriandrum sativum)** bear in mind that there are those loyal to the tender young leaves of coriander (like slugs) and those who would regard it analogous to eating their old slippers. If you're one of those sworn to die by coriander then enjoy it in salad, curries, Thai and Mexican food, sauces and rice dishes. It is an appetite stimulant and also reduces flatulence. Use of this herb is dated as far back as the ancient Egyptians, found in Tutankhamun's tomb. Turn salads and other meals into a spicy affair with a load of coriander; Egyptians swore by its aphrodisiac qualities! (Perhaps that's why there are so many slugs in my garden!)

The kingly **basil (Ocimum basilicum)**, how could we neglect the toss of the regal leaf into the salad bowl, with or without a petrified slug clinging to it? Unfortunately too many swear allegiance to sweet basil when so many interesting varieties are available; amongst them are cinnamon (O.b.'cinnamon'), lemon (O.b. citriodorus), green ruffles (O.b. 'green ruffles'), bush basil (O.b. var. minimum), greek, (O.b. var. minimum 'greek'), etc.

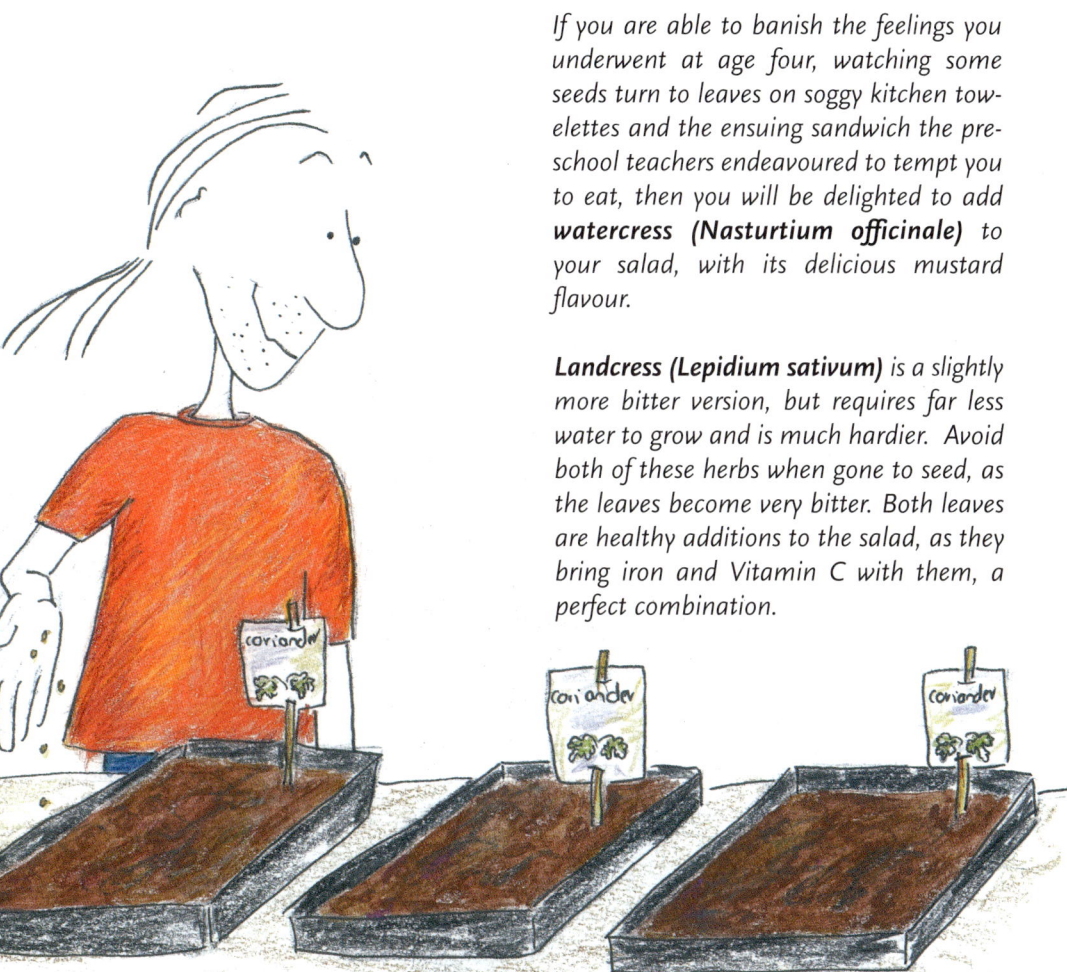

Ask ... your local slug population.

If you are able to banish the feelings you underwent at age four, watching some seeds turn to leaves on soggy kitchen towelettes and the ensuing sandwich the pre-school teachers endeavoured to tempt you to eat, then you will be delighted to add **watercress (Nasturtium officinale)** to your salad, with its delicious mustard flavour.

Landcress (Lepidium sativum) is a slightly more bitter version, but requires far less water to grow and is much hardier. Avoid both of these herbs when gone to seed, as the leaves become very bitter. Both leaves are healthy additions to the salad, as they bring iron and Vitamin C with them, a perfect combination.

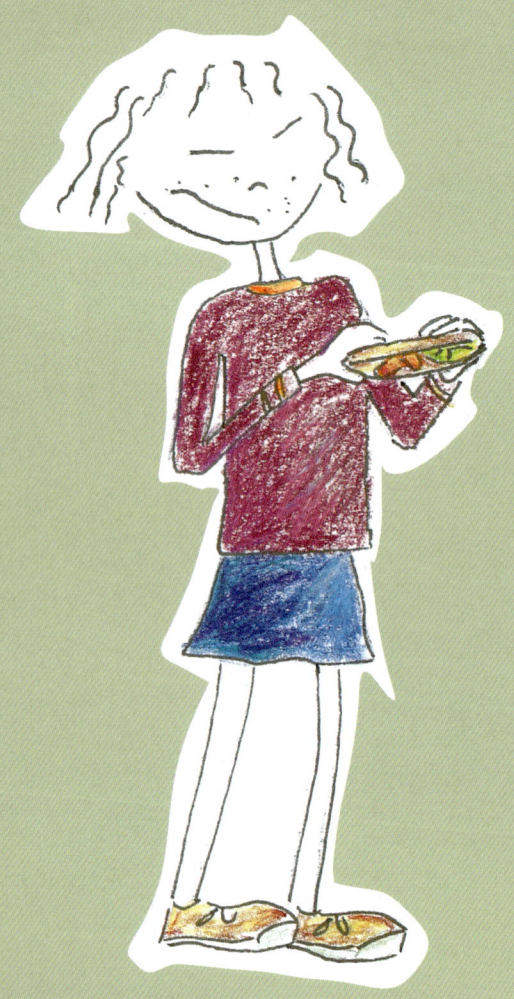

Be very quiet when harvesting **Vietnamese coriander (Plygonum odoratum).** This stealthy green leaf, with a red bite, is certain to attract the attention of slugs as both relish boggy conditions. New to our gardens and tastebuds, this herb came via Australia's Vietnamese immigrants and has spread like wild chilli. Go easy on it in salads, as it has the veneer of a well mannered, lemon-flavoured leaf, but with the tendency to about-turn and bite back. Try a pinch of young leaves in your salads and a handful thrown over Asiatic food or on hot meals on those chilli-less days. Take care that this colonist does not follow you to your salad bowl, creeping into all the rich, moist areas of your garden and annihilating the native species.

Whilst dutifully weeding your garden, be sure to keep the kitchen window open and practice your aim of the **dandelion (Taraxacum officinale)** leaves into the salad bowl. As well as bringing a new meaning to tossing the salad, it is a plant friendly to your digestive system and rich in Vitamins A, B, C and D. The tastiest are the young leaves, which can be picked from the centre of the plant, rather than the older, more bitter leaves. For some or other reason slugs tend to leave these alone, and that perhaps is why it is a weed ...

FURTHER ADDITIONS

Yes, yes, let loose on the slugs with gay abandon just to be able to add that extra bite ...
Calendula leaves, marjoram, chives, French tarragon, thyme, savoury, garlic chives, shallots

FLOWERS FOR SALADS

Calendula, violet, lavender, bergamot, borage, jasmine, hyssop, basil, nasturtium

things that go crunch in the night...

There are things that crunch and sup all night,
To reveal a morning's war torn sight,
Stalks derobed of appendaged leaves,
And seedlings left with a silver path, that weaves,
through beds of lettuce and dismembered peas:
even a hardened gardener falls to her knees.
Such carnage incites Iris to nuke her garden,
But she cannot poison as well as pardon.
If you ask, what troubles or what ails?
She replies, "Those slugs and housebound snails!
They've decimated all my new born basil"
Gone are the eyes that held the gardener's dazzle!

It is night! Iris, pyjamed, descends from the porch,
rooted with wellies, empowered with a torch, gliding snails know not what is at stake.
The moon flinches, the plants awake, at the screams of adjacent plants' demise,
the steady devouring, piece by piece.

Fear not! Wild Iris arrives as saviour to all,
from comfrey, large to basil, small.

The snails detect a trembling earth
of Iris nearing, beset by gardener's mirth.
Alas, nature forgot to equip escargot to flee,
Their caravans exposed for all to see,
Zap! The torch illuminates,
As Iris alters their course of fate!
Crunch! The sound of snailish squish,
Iris, natural gardener, evolves a sadistic niche!

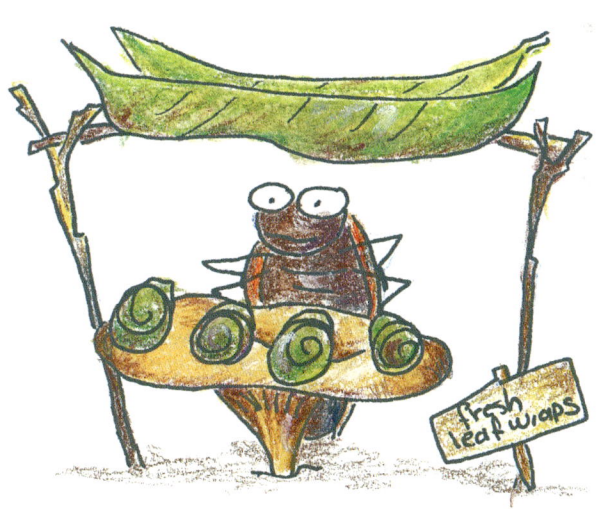

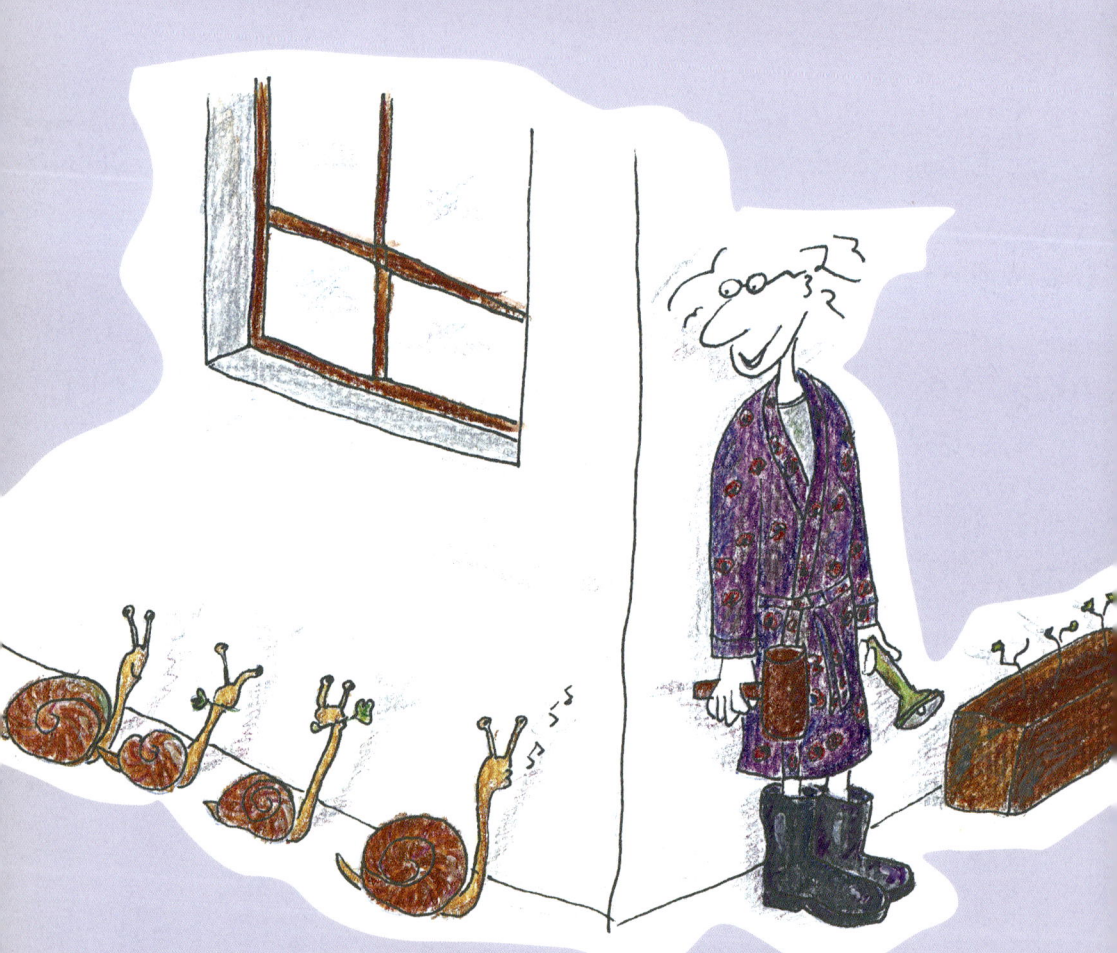

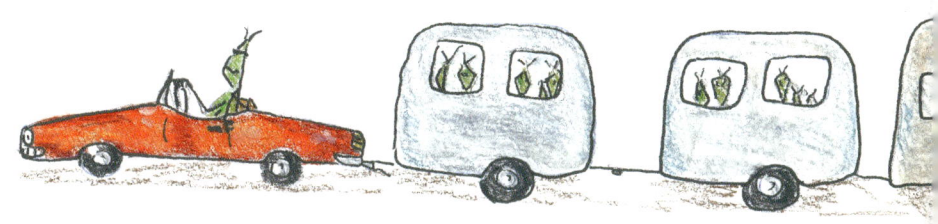

Oh, the despair of the gardener, as clans of snails, slugs, grasshoppers, caterpillars, cutworms etc move into your garden, establishing a chain of 24 hour fast food outlets. Fortunately, nature provides the best solution in destroying this cartel, in the form of the *insect mafia*, who parade your grounds mercilessly, indulging in acts of cannibalism, blood sucking and guerrilla warfare, as they clean out these food halls. This is your trump card in nature, often euphemistically referred to as an ecosystem.

There are times, however, when the chemical war takes its toll on these Mafioso, and we are compelled to call in the superhero herbs, in order to put an end to this free-for-all banquet. Be warned, this chapter is not for the queasy ...

THINGS THAT GO CRUNCH IN THE NIGHT ...

On occasion I have shared a disquieting meal with indelicate salad eaters, but that is nothing in comparison to the sounds of herbivorous diners crunching in your garden. The acute hearing of a dog would be a gardener's nightmare and would surely see mental institutions overflowing with them! Contemplate the agony of lying awake at night, listening to the sound of a tribe of snails annihilating your American brown lettuce, the rapid crunch on your baby basil or the cold calculating slither of a slug towards your freshly planted rocket. The mere thought can make the 8 o'clock news seem palatable in comparison.

Before you rush off for tranquillisers, you can relax, as there are traps, tricks and beguiling ways to lure slugs and snails to their death, terrorising these spineless creatures. **Your first attempt in snail culling would be to create a snail beer hall in your garden.** *Do this by pouring some beer into cut off yoghurt cups and bury these half way into the soil. The trick is to only half fill the cup, so that the mucous heads overdo it in their zest to get to the beer, fall in and drown in their gluttony.*

If beer is too good to waste on the perpetrators of botanical infanticide, try the eggshell approach, but be sure to keep an eye on your cholesterol levels as you eat your way through omelettes, scrambled egg, creme brulee, egg custard etc. in order to acquire a sufficient eggshell hoard. Sprinkle these thickly around your plants to create an unpleasant road to paradise and the lettuce leech is forced to seek greener pastures. (Perhaps your neighbours'?)

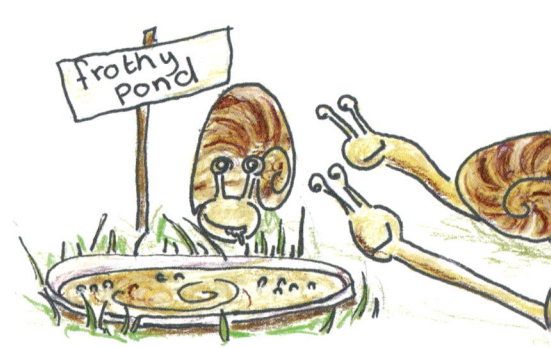

My ova-vegetarian and teetotaler friends have surely hurtled to the next chapter, which is unfortunate, as there is a gentler option:

> Soak a head of garlic in cold water (about one litre), leave this overnight and then strain. Add some dish-washing liquid to this (to make it stick) and spray on your dainties at least twice a day. As with all home-made methods, persistence is required.

For those less interested in egg dishes, the odour of garlic and fishing inebriated snails out of flat beer, there is, of course, the torch and large wellingtons method ...

As for the well lubricated relatives, slugs, who, like you, are fond of rich and fertile gardens, mulching with wood ash will cause their demise. The ash causes them to secrete more mucous to the point of exhaustion and yes, sadly, death.

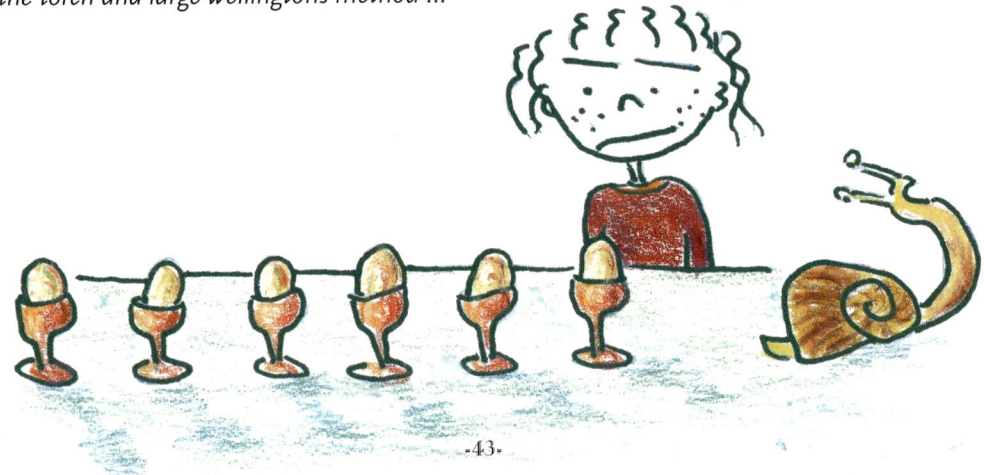

Prevention is after all the preferred method. In order to keep snail and slug populations down, eliminate the dark, damp areas in your garden where these creatures set up their own dens of iniquity. (And we know what that does for family planning.) Fortunately nature also has its controls, so welcome birds and other predators into your garden by planting a diverse selection of plants and shrubs. Many of them are escargot connoisseurs and even slugs themselves place snail eggs on their menu. The larvae of many insects too eat slugs and snails, so kindly think before you squish.

● MORE THINGS THAT GO CRUNCH …

It's hard not to have a soft spot for velvety caterpillars. The bigger they get the more difficult it is to squash these mobile Matisse-like canvases; after all, caterpillars are merely prepubescent butterflies. These creatures, however, are the 'eat as much as you like' garden restaurant patrons and getting rid of them is about as easy as dealing with barflies at closing time. Wormwood, fortunately, will come in handy here and a spray can be made as follows:

> wormwood spray:
>
> Take a bucket, fill it with wormwood leaves and cover with water. Leave overnight. Strain. Add squirt of soap. Dilute 1:10 and spray. Keep remainder of potion in fridge.

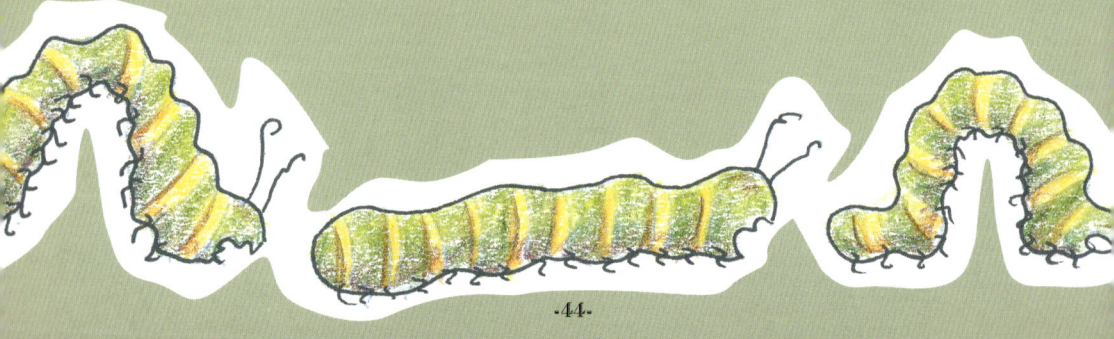

WASPS ...

For lazy gardeners, it is convenient to enlist the services of the insect guerrillas, namely wasps. These aviators paralyse their prey through stinging them and proceeding to lay their eggs on the mummy. The eggs take a few weeks to hatch on the caterpillar and then voila - instant fresh larva food. Other than caterpillar, wasp infant formula comes in a variety of flavours viz. fly, beetle, grasshopper, spider, aphid and cutworm. (Well, Nestlé isn't quite an option in the insect kingdom!)

CUTWORMS ...

Discovering plants devoured by cutworms is somewhat like returning home after a burglary; there's a noticeable absence of both possessions and the perpetrator. The same can be said of the devoured plant and its eater. If you dig around the base of the plant you may find the cutworms but that is tantamount to catching the thief once your DVD player is engulfing someone else's cinematic preferences.

Once again prevention is best, particularly as once they've finished their meal there is no cure. So protect delicate seedlings by placing yoghurt cups, with their bottoms cut out, around the plants. At times the ratio of plant victims to your yoghurt appetite is too big. This recipe will give cutworms their just desserts. No, it certainly is not kind, but necessary.

cutworm straightjacket recipe:

Make a mixture of molasses, sawdust and wheatbran. Place it around their evening meal. They wallow in their pudding, which stiffens and prevents mobility, creating a king of cutworm éclair for birds and other predators.

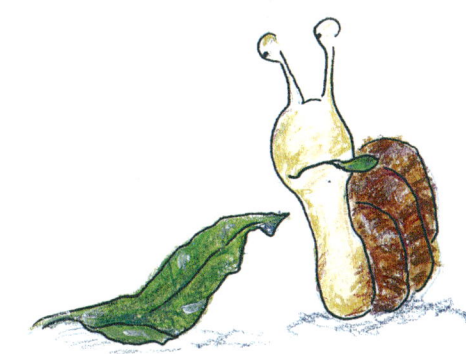

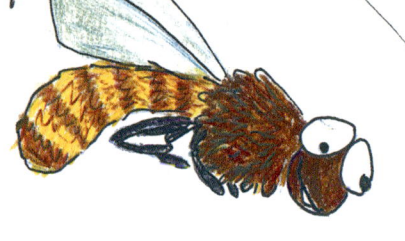

THINGS THAT GO ZZZ IN THE NIGHT ...

It is summertime, you are being attacked by grumpy matrons on night duty, with oversized syringes embedded in their heads, you awake, only to discover that you're being consumed by mosquitoes. In such times a roll in the pennyroyal can be of greater benefit than a roll in the hay, but if you have no one to frolic with, then you can rub pennyroyal onto your skin to ward off these bad tempered bloodsuckers. However, if you are caught with your pants down, pennyroyal can also ease the itch of the bites. Interestingly, it is only the female that sucks blood, which she needs to produce eggs. The males prefer the softer option of vitamin packed plant juice. In order to be really prepared for these bad tempered ovulators make an oil from all or some of these mozzie deterrents - pennyroyal, southernwood, basil, lemongrass (citronella). (See chapter on oils.)

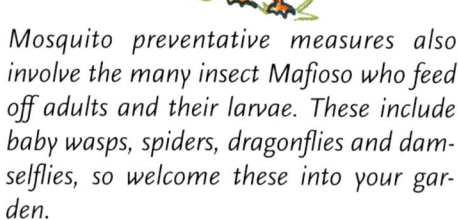

Mosquito preventative measures also involve the many insect Mafioso who feed off adults and their larvae. These include baby wasps, spiders, dragonflies and damselflies, so welcome these into your garden.

THINGS THAT GO BZZ IN THE DAY ...

I find bees to be such saucy insects, dabbling around in plants' sexual organs so unashamedly, dashing to whichever flower displays its wares most seductively. Such brazen creatures are best left alone; however, if one does happen to commit suicide on your person, lavender oil is a most soothing solution. See 'things that go itch in the night' for more kamikaze victim remedies.

Another potential pest is the ant. Normally found in poor soil, ants can be beneficial as they aerate and turn the soil. Should they become a problem in your garden you can add compost and they should get the hint; only to reappear in your sugar bowl. Watching them get away with consuming all that sugar with no side effects, is almost sufficient reason to engage in chemical warfare. However, where ants truly become problematic in the garden is when they become taxis for aphids, scale or mealy bug, setting up diner populations on the next plant. The ants seek out the sweet secretions these pests secrete (some creature will resort to any means for a fix!) and they in turn hitch a ride to the next settlement. Insects always presume life is greener on the other side and after they have finished with one plant, it certainly is!

Troublesome ants can be disposed of by a combination of equal parts borax and icing sugar. Leave it around their routes, where they will find it and transport it back to their holes, inducing underground genocide.

This is not damaging to the environment, but I would not suggest sprinkling it on your cornflakes!

For pacifists, pennyroyal and tansy can be used as deterrents, by placing it around their holes. You can also rub pennyroyal across your kitchen floor for a similar effect.

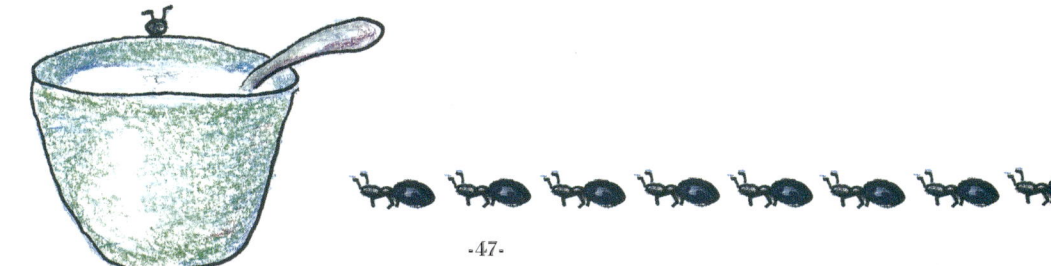

As for the other pesties involved in this crime syndicate, such as scale, mealy bug and aphids, they can be suffocated with a solution of soapy water. Scale might be a bit harder to annihilate. Spray them with an oil such as oleum or linseed, but hopefully the ladybirds and lacewings will get there before you. A fermented nettle spray can control problems with black fly (black aphids). (See teas)

Nematodes! Explorations into the underground network may reveal these entities dining on plants' roots; tomatoes and potatoes being the top of the list of delicacies. What nematodes most dislike (and not surprisingly) are marigolds. Plant these ugly ducklings around your garden to control the nematode population. Marigold roots secrete a substance causing the nematode eggs to hatch, but fail to provide a food source for them. Being sloth -like creatures they cannot travel fast enough to the nearest fast food joint and, well, the rest is history.

THINGS THAT GO SLOSH IN YOUR JUICER ...

This recipe is for when you're really out of your depth. It is not recommended for either Buddhists, Jainists or other pacifists.

Collect about half a cup of the culprit and put them in a blender with two cups of water. Blend. (You may want to close your eyes at this point.) Strain (with your nose blocked) through muslin or an old stocking. Add 1/4 cup of juice to four litres water. Spray onto the victims. Try the following in your bug soup: aphids, pill bugs, bean beetles, cutworm, stinkbugs, armyworm and slugs (I dare you...)

Whatever is left over can be kept in the freezer but be sure you do not confuse it with your frozen veggie soup!

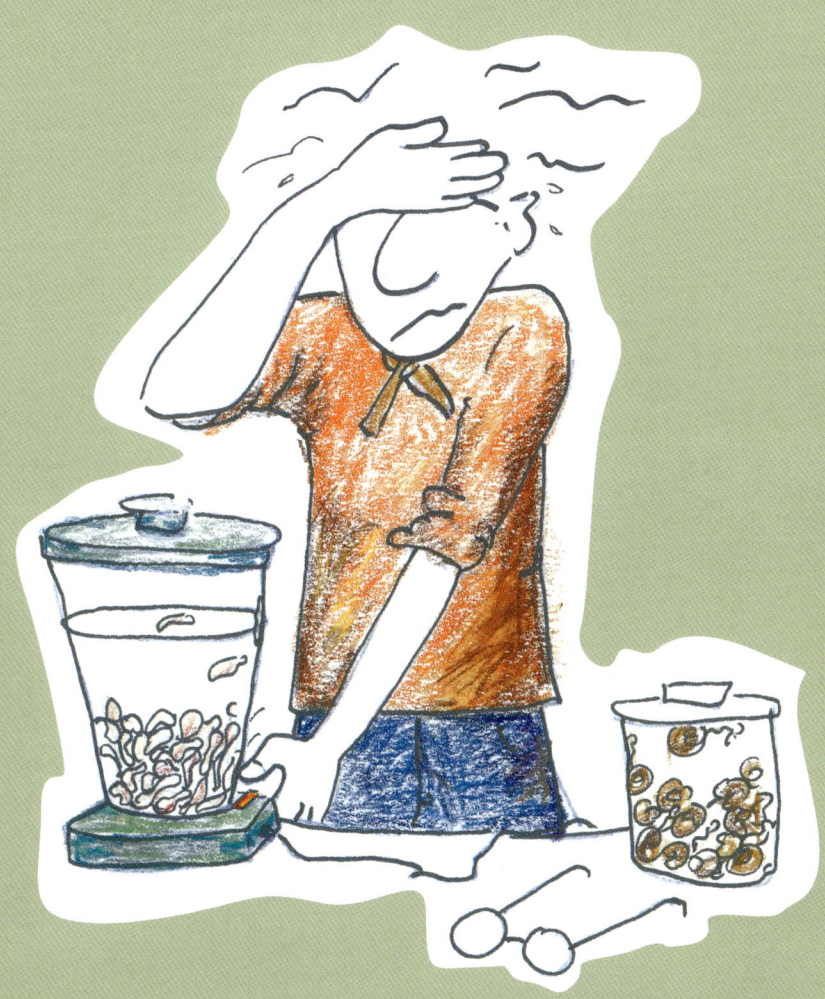

THINGS THAT GO ITCH IN THE NIGHT ...

If you, rather than your plants, have been nominated meal of the day, grasp whichever of the following herb is closest: houseleek, bulbinella (highly recommended), lemon balm (contains an anti-oxidant which reduces inflammation), ribwort and self heal (act as antidotes), freshly sliced onion, calendula, chamomile, lavender and tea tree. A good combination to use in tincture form is thyme, nettle, fennel leaves and seeds and rosemary. A tincture of stinging nettle is highly recommended for urticaria and a concoction that once brought me much needed relief from a terrible rash was a combination of oats, comfrey and nettle. Make a tea from the herbs, add it to raw oats and leave it in the fridge - the coolness is bliss on a hot itchy rash.

THINGS THAT GO SHHH OUT OF YOUR SPRAYER ...

A well-used plant for insect control is pyrethrum (tanecetum cinerariifolium). This is non-toxic to mammals and does not accumulate in the environment or in the bodies of animals. In fact, it can kill pests living on the skin of humans and animals. It works by paralyzing the nervous system of insects. Be aware that it is not selective about who it dishes this treatment out to and may kill beneficial insects. Thus use only when all else has failed and spray at dusk to prevent killing pollinating insects, as it decomposes in bright sunlight.

To make the spray : Add 28g pyrethrum powder to 28ml meths and dilute in 14l water. Spray. The powder can be made out of the dried flowers if you are able to find the plant at your nursery.

THINGS THAT GO MUNCH IN YOUR WOOLIES ...

In between sorting out insect and plant feuds you may return to the comforts of your home to find other creatures have invited themselves to join you in your leisure. Fish moths may have taken to your woolies, and taken a fair share of them. Placing either lavender or southernwood in between layers of clothes will sort out their fashion temptations. You can also make sachets with equal combinations of southernwood, wormwood, lavender and mint (all dried) to place in your wardrobe. Other than the fabric fundis, you may also encounter a couple of bookworms who take the pleasure of your reading matter further than suits you. Placing southernwood between pages, or books in the bookshelf will send them elsewhere for their literary education.

Further afield in your kitchen, you may chance upon weevils residing in your larder. Try placing bay leaves in your dried food to assist them in avoiding temptation. Bay also acts as a preservative.

THINGS THAT TAKE AGES ...

When you have tired of evicting unwanted garden tenants, bear in mind that an organic garden takes a minimum of three years before an ecosystem evolves. In the meanwhile, keep composting and grow a diversity of plants, invest in a recliner, sit back with a gin and tonic and wait ...

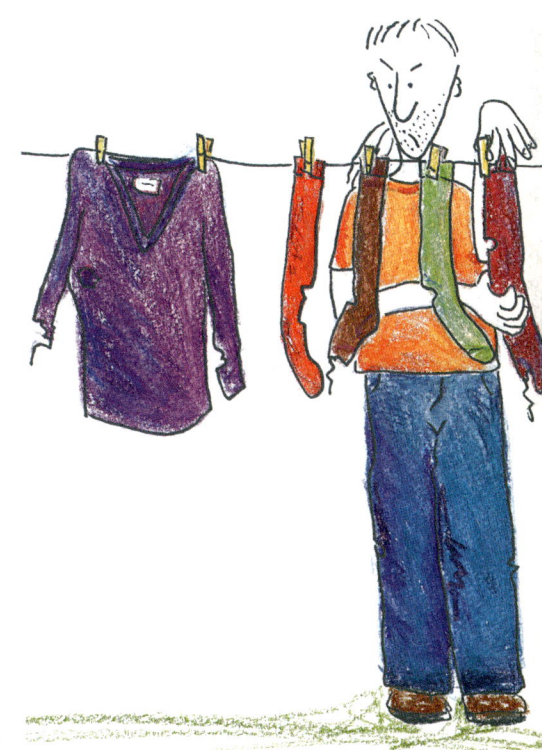

HERBS FOR PESTIES

PEST	HERB
ants	spearmint, tansy, pennyroyal
aphids	nasturtium, spearmint, stinging nettle, southernwood, garlic
black fly	stinging nettle
white cabbage butterfly caterpillar	sage, rosemary, hyssop, thyme, mint, wormwood, southernwood
cutworm	oakleaf mulch, tanbark
flies	oakleaf mulch, tanbark
mosquito	rue, tansy, wormwood, basil
moths	wormwood, southernwood, rosemary, sage, santolina, lavender, mint
slugs	oakleaf mulch, tanbark
weevils	garlic, bay
woolly aphids	nasturtium
nematode	calendula, marigold
squash bugs	tansy
carrotfly	wormwood

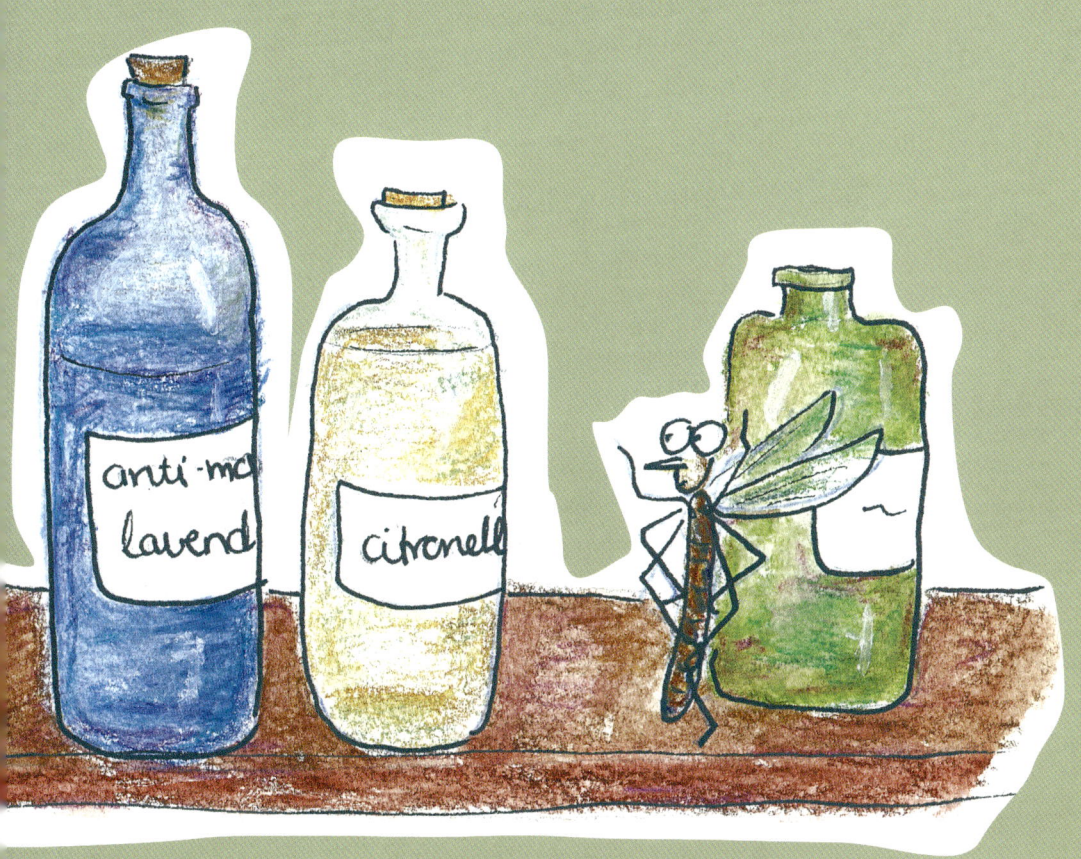

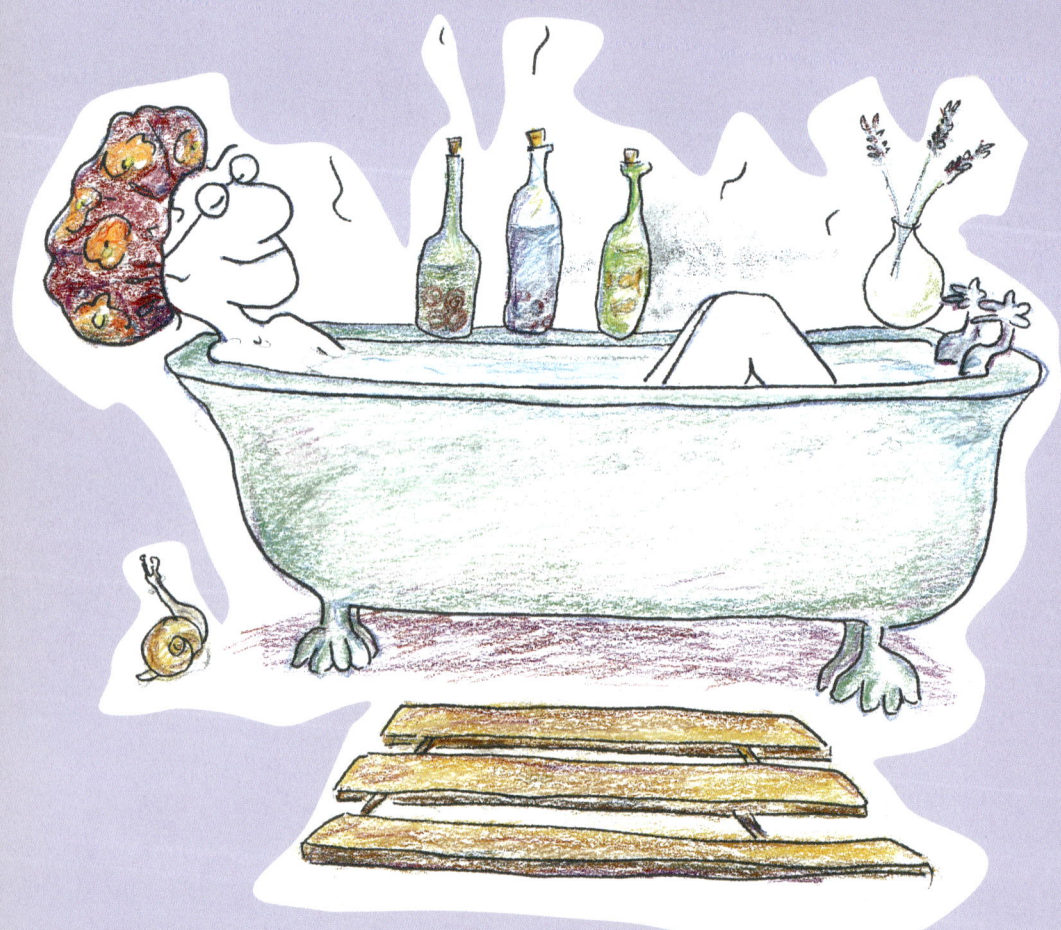

a nasal symphony

Iris takes her body and her nose,
to a bath of herbal oils, to dispose,
of any remnant of crunch or snail,
(the thought no longer leaves her pale),
the stars awake, the moon in shock,
the world still breathes the nightime clock,
as Iris slips into an aromatic oil,
to rid the midnight garnering of soil.

Lavender to calm and chamomile for nerves,
geranium soaks into her gardener's curves.
She delves into her herbal mags,
needing neither wine nor fags,
Iris gardener is quite content,
to live her life within a herbal scent.

Ah, the awe of our schnozzles, that *evolution has somehow left, plonked, right in the centre of our faces, in various sizes and shades. Love your profile or love your cosmetic surgeon, the symphony of the nose is nothing to be sniffed at. No, not with the resident tens of millions of neurons eagerly urging memories and sensations to burst from hidden grey matter crevices, sending either sonatas of warmth to our stomachs or else the spin of the Ferris wheel in your tummy.*

The nose is not all nostalgia, however, as it is connected to the limbic area of the brain where emotions, learning and memory take place. **This section of the brain is like an operator who, once it has received a nasal message, calls various parts of your body, such as your heart, blood pressure, lungs and of course sexual parts, to react.** *The result is countless calls being made merely from the whiff of someone's scent; no wonder we get a few crossed lines now and then.*

With our wonderful protuberances, we love to smell the necks of babies and inhale their sweetness (preferably when they don't smell of Parmesan cheese or overdue nappies), but we're often not too certain about our own necks, let alone the parts attached. How often does anyone ever pass you by and remark on your delicious scent, when you haven't doused yourself with something from the cosmetic industry? Admittedly we cannot repeatedly waft out of an essential oiled bathroom, but herbal bath oils can prolong our 'ooh' aroma for a good length of time. And if there's no one to stick their nose into your neck, or massage you into sweetness, bath oils are great for self-therapy, anti-stress and simple self-indulgence.

Many plants are in agreement with us about wanting to smell good and do a much better job of it too. They manufacture their delights inside petals, bark, resin, peels, roots or leaves. These essential oils are persuaded out of their hidey cells by processes of distillation, expression, enfleurage or by means of a solvent. This practice would require conversion of one's greenhouse into a laboratory, so it is best left to the olfactorily devoted or white-coated people. For our purposes we merely make a diluted version of essential oils, but we can still appear out of the mists of the bathroom refreshed, desirable and soothed, regardless of the shape of our noses.

Herbal oils serve to please more than our smell organs, as we also like to indulge our skin, which we spend a lifetime's fortune on trying to prevent from looking flabby and un-ironed. The skin is also the largest organ of the body, interrelated to our brain and our nervous system, which in turn is hot-wired to the rest of our body. And that is why a good oily bath can leave us feeling like newborn babies.

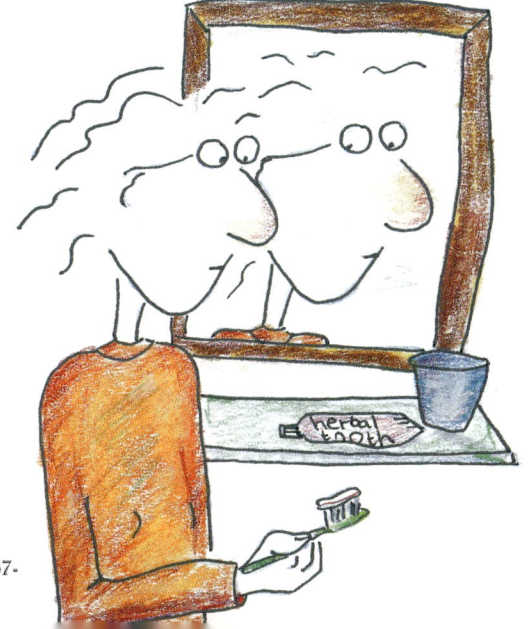

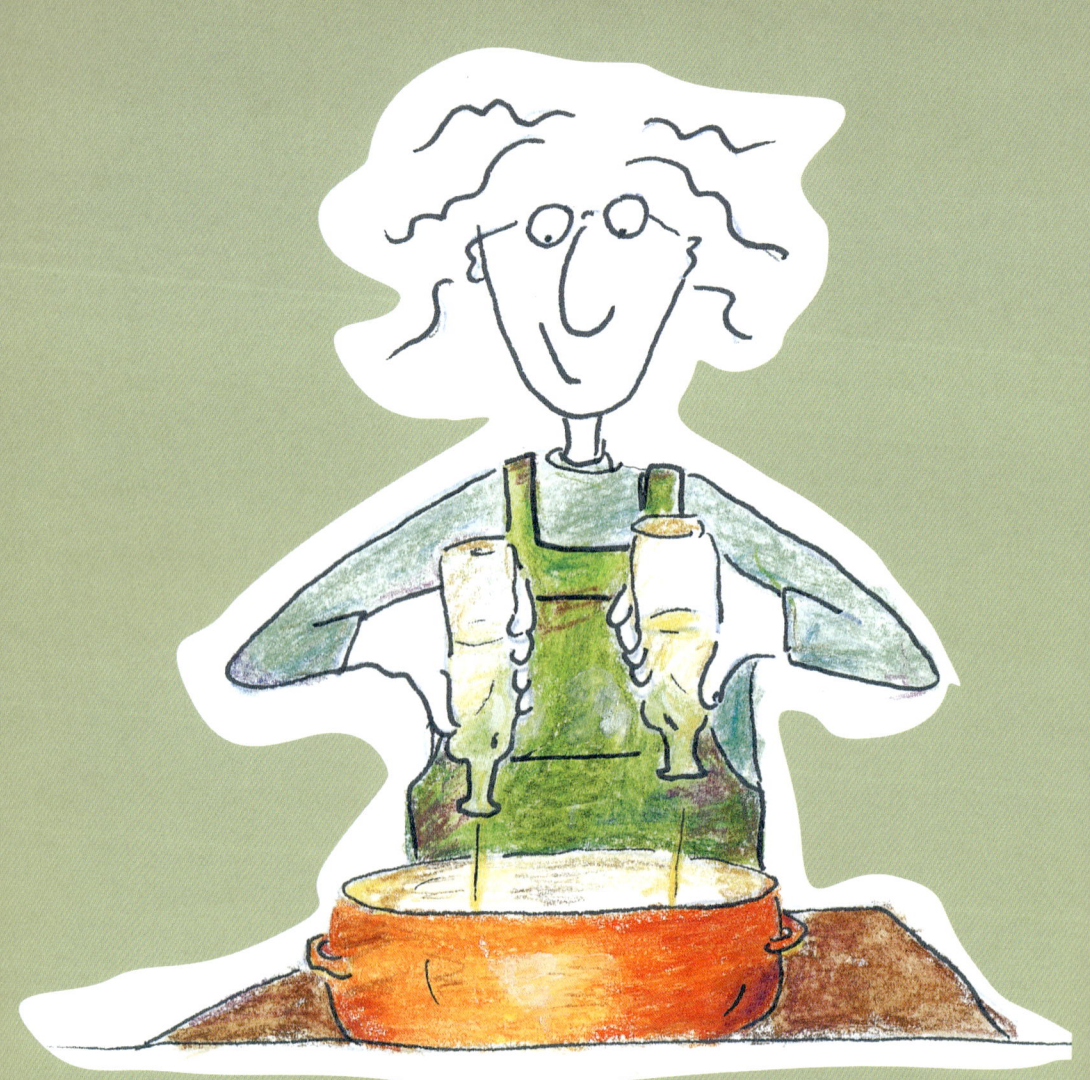

MAKING HERBAL OILS

Producing home herbal oils does not extract as intensively the essential oils within the plant as the procedures employed to coerce essential oil out. This does not mean they are ineffective or that the normal 'be careful of's' do not apply. Firstly, be sure not to use a plant that can affect an underlying health condition adversely, for example a skin or heart condition, blood pressure etc. For safety do not lie in a herbal bath up to the neck or for longer than 20 minutes and do not let the water rise as high as your heart, especially if you have a wobbly heart (and that's not referring to any kind of 'amour' here). Be sure that you know the effects of the plants chosen.

The process:

These oils make excellent gifts, especially when you're stony broke and your Christmas family is boundless. This method can be used for culinary as well as bodily oils; the process is the same. For cooking oils use olive, almond or cold-pressed sunflower oils. Our skins enjoy almond, jojoba, apricot kernel oils etc.

Take a wide-mouthed jar and fill it to capacity with your herb/herbs of your choice. Fill the jar to the brim with oil and close. Leave it in a warm place for about two weeks, turning daily. You can remove the herbs and replace them with fresh ones if you desire a stronger oil. Then strain with muslin into an attractive jar and cork it. Dark bottles or jars work best, otherwise keep the oil out of the light. Wheat germ oil makes a good preservative: pour 1/20th to mixture. In order to satisfy eyes as well as nose, add a few sprigs of herbs, shells, little pebbles, marbles, plastic goldfish, whatever tickles your fancy! Next, run your bath or beckon your masseur closer ... (Don't wallow in your salad oil or massage your lettuce with chamomile oil.)

HERBS TO USE:

For bath/massage oils:

Chamomile - *germicidal, anti-bacterial – skin rashes; add to bath for overwrought nerves*

Sweet Basil - *concentration*

Bergamot - *uplifting*

Roman Chamomile - *relaxing*

Fennel – *anti-toxin*

Hyssop - *sedative*

Juniper - *stimulant*

Lemon Balm - *anti-depressant, relaxant, insomnia, headaches*

Lavender – *soothing, energy, burns, stings, cuts; add to bath to calm irritable children; place on temples to give headache relief. Also useful for inflammation, rheumatic aches, anxiety, insomnia and depression*

Rosemary - *invigorating, anti-bacterial and anti-fungal, helps poor circulation, headaches*

Sweet Marjoram – *calming, relaxing*

Thyme – *stimulant, fungicidal, soothes aching back*

Rose Geranium - *relaxing, pre-menstrual tension, dermatitis, eczema, herpes, dry skin, depression, eczema, rashes*

Peppermint – *massage to relieve muscular pains*

Eau de Cologne Mint - *uplifting*

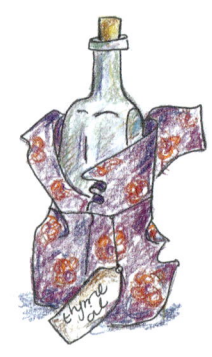

Cooking and salad oil

Herbal oils are excellent for cooking as many herbs have antiseptic and anti-bacterial qualities, making them perfect for preserving. Furthermore many culinary herbs aid digestion and stimulate appetite, not to mention enhance the flavour of food. Herb vinegars can be made by means of the same process, but not exposed to direct sunlight. Be sure not to allow the vinegar to come into contact with metal. Pickling jars work best.

Dribble ...

Thyme (Thymus vulgaris)

Residing inside an infusion of oil is a busy task for thyme as it takes on the chore of breaking down fatty foods. This could almost be an excuse to go overboard with the oil, dripping it onto salads, tomato dishes or steamed vegetables. It is most delicious for dipping ciabatta into, or used in a marinade for meat or vegetables.

Chives (Allium schoenoprasum)

Another herb seeking longevity is chives, as it becomes scarcer during winter. Chives work best in an oil or vinegar when accompanied by other herbs, but its whole leaves and flowers make an attractive display in the bottles. When not pouring onto salads, slosh a little oil in the pan to cook egg dishes or trickle over baked potatoes.

Rosemary (Rosemarinus officinalis)

Rosemary is a herb that enjoys scorching in the oven, be it next to lamb, potato, courgettes or other sizzling foods. Keep rosemary oil handy for roasting instead of using the fresh herb for a tempting change. Grilled tomatoes will be delighted by a dressing of this oil, as will kebabs, baked potatoes, baked fish, chicken and beans. Use to braise when starting casseroles and tomato dishes.

Marjoram and oregano (Oreganum sp.)

Marjoram is the better salad oil, as oregano is stronger, but both herb oils should find their way onto Italian dishes, like pizzas and pasta. Don't leave out dousing tomatoes, beans, courgettes and other vegetables.

Basil (Ocimum basilicum sp.)

We all love basil in salads, with tomato, in pasta and on pizza, with rice, in fact with anything. Unfortunately we sadly have to watch its demise as winter beckons. Making an oil from these delicious leaves will enable you to spread the taste through the basil famine, dribbling it on everything including salads, eggplant, marrows, squash, tomatoes, potatoes etc. Recipe: A delicious salad is the traditional Greek with tomato, olives, basil and halved hard boiled egg. Run some basil oil and vinegar over it, even if basil is still in abundance.

Tarragon (Artemesia dracucnulus)

The French tarragon is in all circles considered superior to the **Russian (A. dracunculoides)**, although both hail from Russia. The latter would more aptly be named Siberian, due to its origins and toughness. The French, though frailer, is less bitter, with its sweet anise-like taste, touched with pepper. Indispensable to French cuisine, it joins parsley and chervil in fines herbes, and can be cooked with green beans and other vegetables. It is delicious with poultry, tomatoes (especially stuffed) and rice dishes as well as added to mayonnaise, butter or cream cheese. Other values of tarragon are that it is an appetite stimulant, and digestive aid. Tarragon is another herb that will appreciate bottled immortality, be it in vinegar or oil, as it dies down in winter. Dribble onto avocado, chicken, vegetables, salads etc.

Bay (Laurus nobilis)

Bay is an excellent addition to a herbal oil, especially as it aids digestion as well as being a good preservative. Traditionally bay is used in marinades, and added to soups, stews and curries. Any oil containing bay can substitute for the fresh herb in these and other dishes.

Bay oil can even be added to your bath oil to relieve aching limbs. Take care to test on your skin, as some skins are most irritated by the thought of splashing about in a salad oil, especially one containing bay.

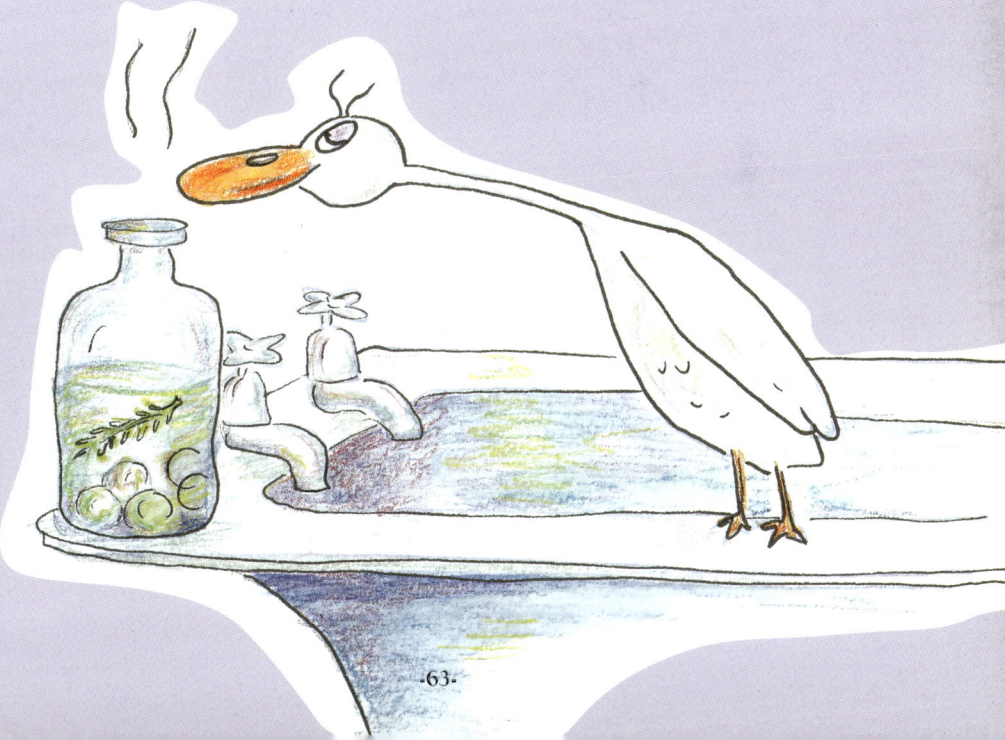

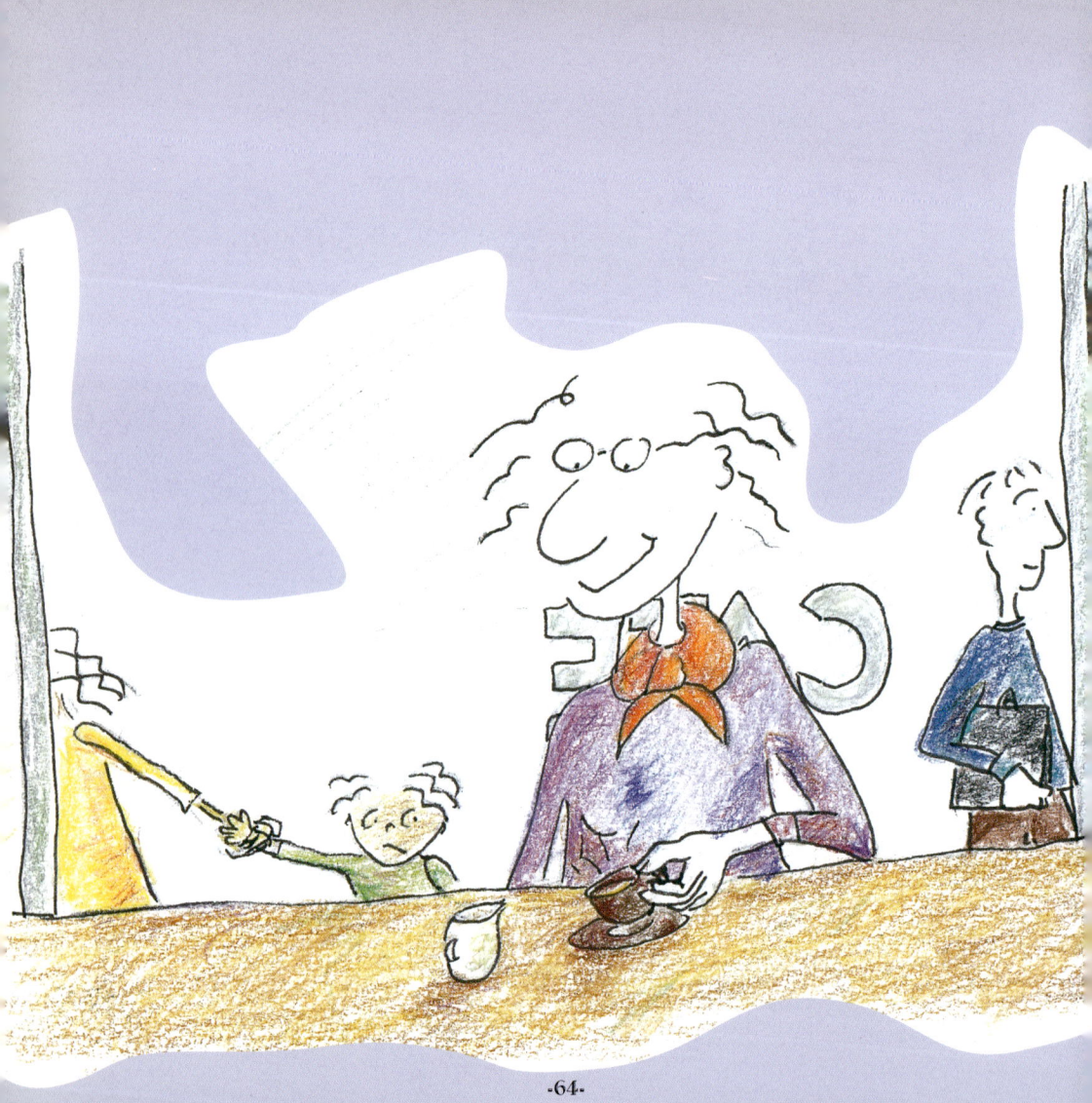

the tea room

Basil slips some chaste tea into his herbal brew
he thinks he has discovered something smart and very new,
his books have recommended this tree for female lust,
but because he was distracted by his pending pelvic thrust,
he failed to notice further down the page,
some info handed down from age to age,

that 'chaste tree', as its name suggests
rids male libido of its zest.

So Basil cannot seem to find
why his diversions are no longer of a dirty mind,

Oblivious, Iris sips her herbal teas,
she knows they help with her arthritic knees,
and doses Angelica for colds and flu,
she'll try anything from old to new,

but on what Iris really depends
is strongly roasted, caffeinated blends!!!!

Prior to Ceylon humans sipped catnip tea. Not quite to your taste? Well, judging by the habits of most tea drinkers anything can taste good if well disguised with a bit of cow and processed sugar cane. However, it is possible to make very delicious teas without these accoutrements. As herbal teas are absolutely tannin and caffeine free you might feel compelled to sneak off for a double espresso round the corner now and then, just to jumpstart your brain!

Now let's get it straight: tea, tisane, decoction or infusion? A tea will have been subject to various degrees of heat to cause fermentation. Even green tea is lightly fermented, although not to the same degree as Ceylon tea. An infusion on the other hand is about the same as a tisane (which relies on less exact measurements) and comes straight from the plant in a fresh or dried form. Hot water is added and it is left to steep, covered, for five to 10 minutes. A decoction, on the other hand, is boiled as harder plant parts are used such as roots or sticks (e.g. licorice or ginger).

As the old adage goes, the worse it tastes, the better it is for you, but let's face it, you have to be very sick to endure drinking some herbal concotions. Fortunately **there are infusions that your taste buds will do the hula hoop for.** Try them on their own or combinations thereof. (In this chapter they are called teas, which make them seem more enticing somehow!)

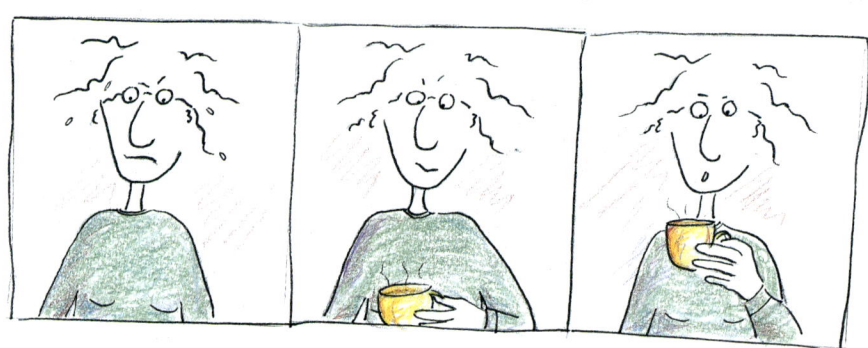

Mint/Peppermint (Mentha x piperita)
This tea is worth making merely to stick your nose into to remind your sinuses that there's more to life than being stuffed up. And then of course you should also drink it, and that is worth being a tastebud for with its delicious and refreshing minty essence. Further down, this zinging tea will encounter your stomach. It may need loads of luck as it enters the land of reconstituted baked beans, oily chips and chocolate mousses. For some reason, unbeknown to non-plants, peppermint will take on this challenge and sort out the resultant gaseous chambers. Not bad for a couple of mentholated leaves. Another plus for peppermint is that it helps concentration and eases headaches.

In my opinion garden or **spearmint (M. spicata)** should stick to peas and lamb, but peppermint was evolved to be brewed. There are a great variety of other minty choices, but stay clear of posh varieties which have a great aroma, but terrible taste. Experiment at your tastebuds' peril, but don't touch **pennyroyal (M. pulegium)**; your kidneys will have you at the doctor for it!

All mints are extremely exuberant growers, which allows you to harvest and dry the leaves for when winter chills cause their enthusiasm to fall a bit flat.

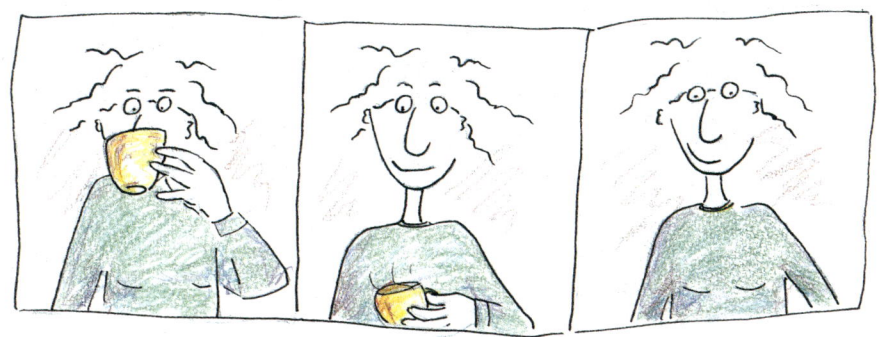

Ginger (Zingiber officinale)

Ginger - no, not the neighbour's orange cat - is another refreshing tea to indulge in, fresh or dried, on its own, or added to other herbal teas. It will definitely get your blood out of the pit stop and back on the track. Sickies will benefit from it, as well as stomachs that are a bit thunder stormish. Those with travel sickness and neo-natal babies wobbling in their tummies will also benefit from its nausea-reducing properties. Being a steamy kind of herb, ginger enjoys growing in the tropics, but can be grown indoors in cooler climates if kept cosy. Ginger's multiplying rhizome will ensure that there is always enough for tea and garden and its beautiful flower will please aesthetically, whilst you brew.

Chamomile (Chamaemelum nobile – Roman, Matricaria recutita – German)

When all the Mr McGregors of the world have run after you, a cup of chamomile tea will put you to rest with its soothing and calming qualities. Furthermore these flowers will calm the Peter Rabbits running around your children's heads or stomachs at night.

What Peter Rabbit's mother will never reveal is that chamomile tea requires a rather large harvest of flowers to keep you going and is best dried before use. Not even Mr McGregor's herbal patch does the trick, so she buys it organically grown from a health shop. Good thinking, Mrs Rabbit.

Chamomile comes in many versions; the two most commonly used are the perennial lawn or roman and the annual German. The most prolific to grow is the German variety, which will self-seed, readily making your tea production a far more abundant affair.

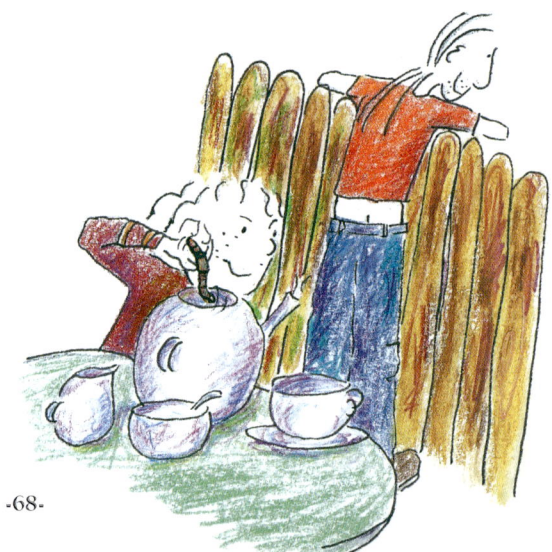

Fennel (Foeniculum vulgare)

All parts of fennel can be sacrificed to the teapot. Decapitate the seed heads and dry them. It will keep fennel population explosions under control and provide instant tea throughout the year. Breastfeeding moms will find this a useful tea, when the dairy's production slumps. It is also useful to ease colicky babies' tummies as well as queasy and bloated adult stomachs. Eyes will be happy to hear of its use as a wash for conjunctivitis and those with liver damage should sip three times a day to repair their wonky livers (especially after excessive alcohol indulgence).

Licorice (Glycyrrhiza glabra)

If you are familiar only with the sticky black plaits lying in wait at your sweet shop, then you will be pleasantly delighted to find that licorice is a plant and the tacky goo derived from it hails from the root. As a tea it will ease sore throats and bronchial catarrh and is also helpful for stomach ulcers. Generally good for anything, just drink it. Grow in a rich, deep, well-cultivated soil. The root can also be bought dried. As with other

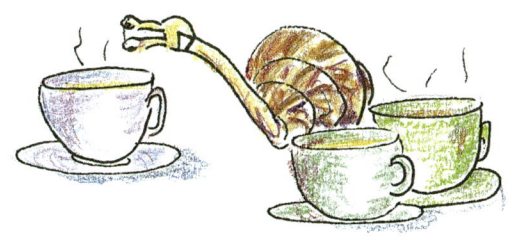

roots, licorice is best boiled, rather than infused.

Bergamot (Monarda didyma)

Oswego tea became the all-American Brew after ditching Ceylon to the sharks at the Boston Tea Party. Don't throw your Ceylon overboard, however, as adding some Bergamot leaves will produce a taste similar to Earl Grey (Earl Grey essentially contains the oil from the Italian bergamot orange, Citrus bergamia). Benefits that are derived from bergamot are easing of nausea, flatulence and insomnia.

Rose-scented Geranium (Pelargonium graveolens and P. capitatum)

Wrongly named geraniums, these plants arrived in England from the Cape in the mid Seventeenth Century to scent ladies' chambers. Of the various differences between geraniums and pelargoniums, the most obvious are the flowers. True geraniums have petals of equal size, whereas the pelargoinums have the three large petals at the top and the 'lip' of two small petals at the bottom. This difference becomes less apparent with the cultivars. There are many different types, but of the tastiest are the two rose scented varieties. Both of them are Old Cape remedies. P.graveolens is used for calming and soothing, a good night time tea, but also excellent for diarrhoea, vomiting and colic. P.capitatum can be used in place of P.graveolens, but will also aid kidney and bladder ailments along with nausea and flatulence.

Lemon is a popular flavouring chosen by many herbs, which enables us to make many revitalising lemony teas. Use them on their own or throw them all together into the teapot.

Lemon Verbena (Aloysia triphylla)

Your grandmother's favourite, a herb reminiscent of many childhoods. Well, granny was onto something (unfortunately not hallucinogenic), popping these leaves into her underwear drawer, when not sipping them in an infusion. Making lemon verbena tea is a fine excuse to wander off to the bush and launch your nose into its fragrance, but remember it is worth drinking too! Not only is it refreshing, but mildly sedative as well as soothing for stuffy noses and chests. Lemon verbena will also aid indigestion and alleviate nausea.

Lemon Grass (Cymbopogon citrates)

This grass was born to brew. Lemon grass grows so ferociously you can keep deleafing it into your teapot. Yet another herb skilled at driving away ailing stomachs and pesty colds, not to mention softening aching heads.

Lemon Balm (Melissa officinalis)

How soooooothing this balm, with a twist of lemon, is. Consider it the 'easy chair' of herbs as it edges your stress away and slowly rescues your head from aches and tension, lullabying you to sleep. Before you forget, lemon balm is also useful for restoring memory loss. Where were we, oh yes, memory loss ... drink this refreshing tea to improve circulation and tone your heart muscles. If the thought of your or someone else's heart gets your blood pressure soaring, sip an infusion of lemon balm to subdue it.

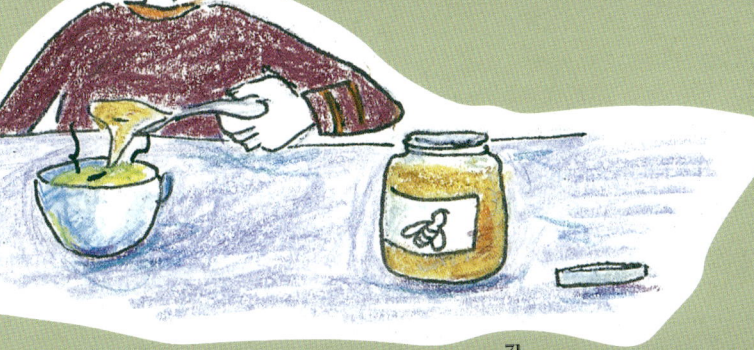

Rooibos Tea (Aspalanthus linearis)

And just when you thought you'd unravelled the tea versus infusion mystery, you are urged to brew up some rooibos tea. This beverage is heat treated and fermented, thereby allowing it to call itself a tea. Originally introduced to the settlers in the Cape Colony by the indigenous people of South Africa, this tea has seeped into teapots world-wide.

Rooibos is a home-bound plant, stubbornly refusing to send its roots into new or foreign terrain, growing only in its natural environment, the Cedarberg area of South Africa. This leaves you to be satisfied with plucking a box from your supermarket shelf, in loose or bagged form. The traditional method of brewing rooibos is by placing the needle-like leaves in a pot and leaving it to simmer very lightly all day, replacing the water as needed. There should always be a pot of rooibos on the go. This robust red African plant does not retire with ease and to many the stronger the brew the tastier, especially as it does not increase in bitterness with prolonged brewing.

Rooibos is the goody-two-shoes of teas, boasting a low tannin content and no caffeine, thus making it suitable for all ages and safe for pregnant women. In South Africa babies are frequently given rooibos to ease colic and many a nappy rash is soothed by an application of cooled tea. Lactating mothers can safely drink rooibos which will stimulate milk flow, ease indigestion and supplement the diet by assisting iron absorption aided by its Vitamin C content. The high mineral content of rooibos makes it helpful in development of good teeth in young children.

For most of us it is too late to change the content of our teeth, but we can employ the help of this tea to allay insomnia, ease skin problems such as acne and eczema, aid digestion and relieve stomach ache. Rooibos is also recommended for the elderly as it stabilises enzyme changes and has an appetite for free radicals. For nervous tension, slip rooibos, rather than yourself, into hot water. Rooibos tea is comfortable hot or cool, in iced tea, in fruit punches, with milk or without, delicious with honey or a slice of lemon. Add other herbal teas to it for added flavour.

Earthworms* are the coffee addicts, but plants incline towards tea. They prefer theirs cool, not iced, and sprayed not poured. The following recipes will give your plants a boost.

(*Sprinkle coffee grounds in your garden to give your earthworms a treat!)

Appease your plants with **chamomile** tea to promote healthy growth and protect against root and soil disease. Another useful plant tea is **dandelion (Taraxacum officinale)**, which, amongst many other nutrients, contains a good supply of copper, for hungry soil. Add to this **stinging nettle (Urtica urens),** which makes plants more resistant to disease and pests. As all of these plants tend towards being weeds you will frequently have sufficient plant food; furthermore, as weeds denude the soil of nutrients, churning them into teas will recycle the goodies.

Chamomile: Take 30g of dried flowers and stand for 24 hours, then strain and dilute in five litres of water. Spray on plants or water soil.

Dandelion: Seep three whole plants in one litre hot water, and cover for half an hour. Strain and use, either as a foliar feed or directly into the ground. This mixture will not store, so use it all at once.

Nettle: Fill a bucket with nettle and cover with water. Leave for a week, strain and spray onto unhappy plants. This spray will also repel aphids.

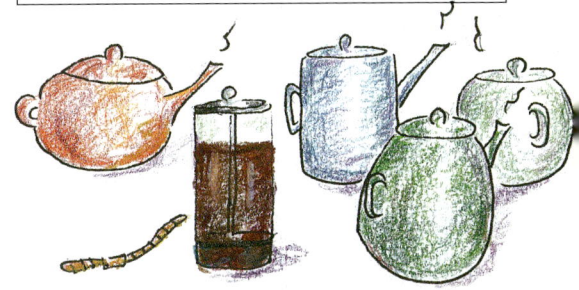

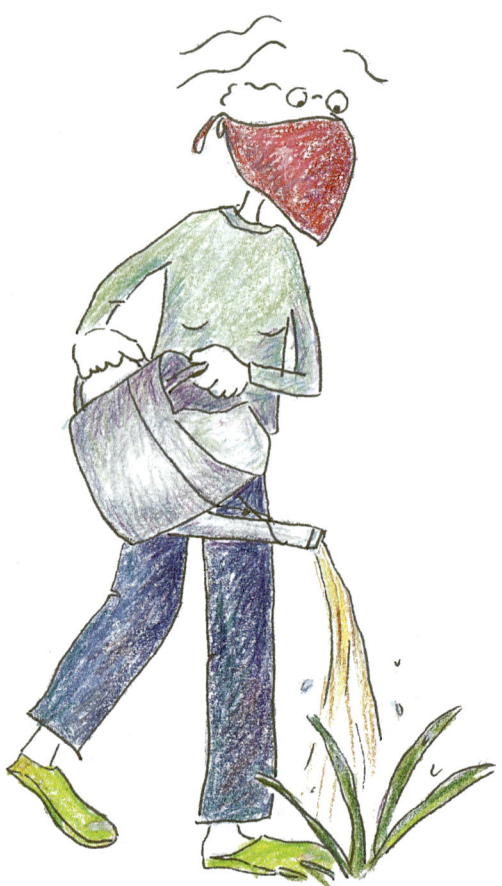

FERMENTED TEAS

Fermented teas are a great hit for plants, even if they are far more odoriferous than our choices of tea. (Although plants may point out that certain of our beverages are fairly pongy too.)

Nevertheless, the following recipes could possibly be managed with one hand. (The other blocking your nose, of course.) It is amazing what some life forms will absorb!

How to go about making dreadfully whiffy comfrey tea:

Well, yes, you'll need some comfrey leaves; pack them into a container and add a little chicken manure to activate it. Cover. After about two to three weeks they will have rotted to an unfriendly smelling brown liquid. Dilute it 1:10 and water your plants with it, or spray as foliar feed. Some recipes recommend placing the mixture in a bucket with holes and this within another bucket. When the potion is ready, you can drain it through into the bottom bucket without splashing any slime onto your linen trousers!
Fermented comfrey tea is rich in potassium and nitrogen, protein, potash, trace elements and minerals. These benefit plant

health and promote a strong cell structure, making them more resistant to disease. Use this tea on all plants, but tomatoes, potatoes, gooseberries, beans and other potash-hungry crops desire it the most. Comfrey tea will also prevent attack by fungi and many insects. (Can't say I blame them!)

A beneficial addition to this recipe is comfrey's cousin **borage (borago officinalis)**, which contains abundant nitrogen, loved by brassicas and melons in particular.

Another fermented tea for plant mollification is the following calendula potion:

> Take 250g calendula flowers to 250ml water. Leave covered for two weeks, to allow fermentation. Strain. Dilute to a 1:10 solution and then spray.

This plant tea will help the growth of healthy plants, making them more resistant to disease. It also strengthens tissues and as an anti-fungal will prevent seedlings from being zapped by damping off disease.

Once again nettle enters the bucket: Use the same quantities as the previous recipe, but leave to ferment for three weeks. This spray will promote plant growth and health, as well as assist it in unhealthy conditions such as drought.

COMPOST ACTIVATORS

On the subject of potentially odorous matter, plants such as calendula, comfrey and nettle make excellent compost activators. Add to this list yarrow, valerian and oak bark. Nettle in particular breaks down to a rich and pleasant humus and can be used as a mulch. Remember that healthy plants need good soil.

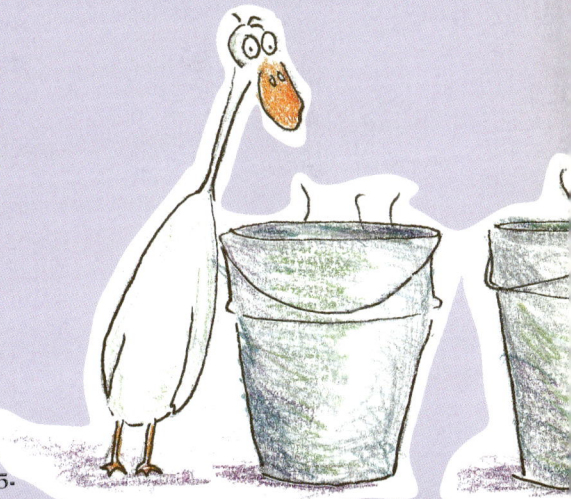

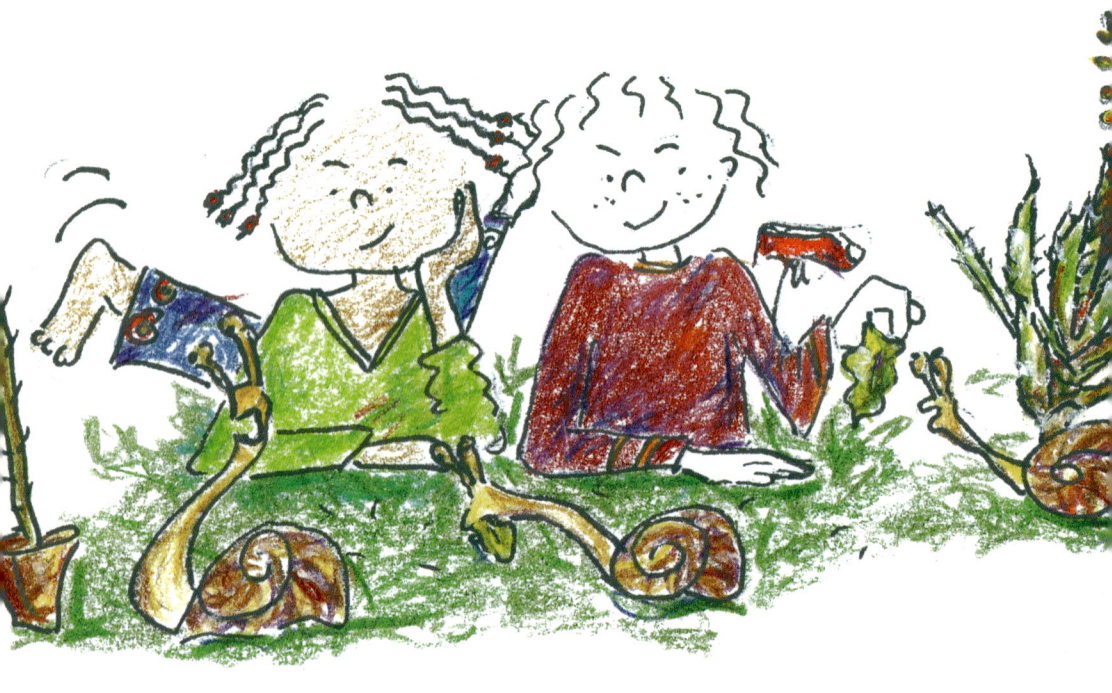

gardens for wild things

You may have spotted Angelica's
penchant for snails,
She picks them up and transports them
in slimy silver pails.

This hobby can suit a young gardener well,
But such an occupation is a mother's hell.
For in Angelica's corner no lushness can be seen,
And her choice is something on which snails are never keen,
For cacti will not be eaten, not spikes nor thorns and pokes.
For Iris it is a tasteless, scentless joke.

Yet snails creep out when least expected,
And Angelica runs, the pest undetected,
She slips, collides and clearly lands
On spikes and thorns on knees and hands,

Her hobby has caused her own demise.
yet to her rescue an anxious mother flies!

That very distinctive flower, lovingly enticed to withdraw from its hiding place and bear its inner blossom to you: the gardener ... and then, snap, your entire raison de jardenner is plummeted before your very soil-tainted eyes ...The culprit: ... your own human seedling.

The worst is that there is no cure for this malaise, only a patient sentinel of the garden as the years mature. In the meantime, we can only attempt to channel the destructive forces into a particular area, for their own selective plucking. This comes with no guarantees, but it does serve to appease the parental guilt for placing nature above nurture. However, soccer balls, thumping boots, 'actionmen' forts and miniature landscapers are beyond any gardener's expertise. When all else fails seek out some new age philosophy, certainly not gardening periodicals or parenting manuals.

Children who have successfully mastered the art of placing a seedling right way up in the ground, without altering its structure too severely, will love to help you make a garden for them. In my experience seeds don't really work until children are old enough to have mastered the art of watering, rather than bathing seeds and their offshoots. In the meantime plant a child's garden around a sand pit or splash pool, under a tree house or with a swing. Children will also relish their own spot in the vegetable or herb bed.

Herbs, in particular, are excellent choices for children's gardens; particularly those that can be felt and smelt. Being natural foragers children also enjoy flowers and plants that can be eaten.

Plant ...

Lamb's Ear (Stachys lanata) - *you will find not only children, but adults too, caressing the silvery-grey rabbit-like ears of this plant. An unusual ground cover with small lilac flowers in summer and a good substitute for a pet!*

Lavender (Lavendula sp.) - *undoubtedly one of the favourites for scent and flowers. Make lavender basket and pillows with children.*

Rosemary (Rosmarinus oficinalis) - *for scent and flowers many children refuse any delicacy with the faintest twig of green in it, but these rosemary biscuits have fooled even the diehard difficult eaters.*

● LAVENDER AND ROSEMARY BISCUITS

360g flour, 250g butter, 100g sugar, milk, twigs of rosemary and lavender leaves

Cream the butter and sugar together and then sift in the flour. Add chopped lavender and rosemary, and mix (You can also do half/half). Knead the dough adding small amounts of milk to create a firm, but rollable dough. Roll about 3mm thick, cut with favourite biscuit cutters and place on greased tray. Bake for 10-15 minutes at 200°C, gas 6, 400°F.

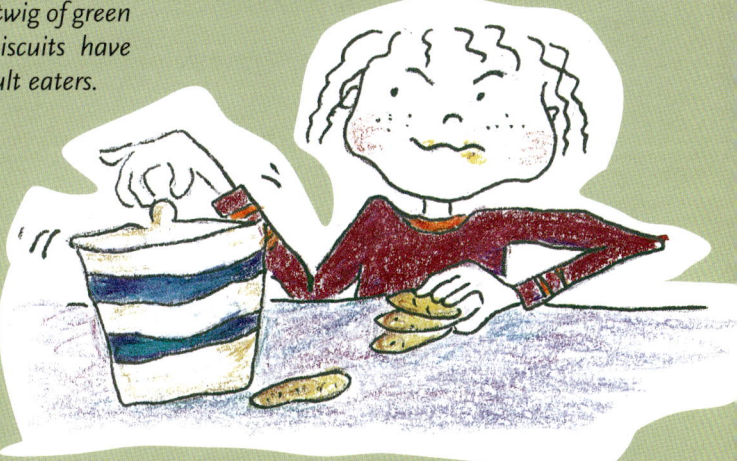

Pelargoniums (Pelargonium so.) - the most delicious aromas that waft from these leaves are matched by the attractive flowers, which are always in abundance, very necessary in a picking garden.

Chamomile - the German species is best, as the lawn chamomile is asking for disaster when the flowers entice bees, who meet the bare feet of summer.

Mint (Mentha sp.) - for compulsive pickers, making soups and cakes in the garden, mint will tirelessly continue its growth, unperturbed.

Angelica - another chewable stem, which can be taken on journeys to alleviate travel sickness.

Calendula – whatever orange flowers remain can be made into a tincture or cream, for those all too frequent cuts, grazes and sores.

Bulbinella (Bulbine frutescens) - children will be lured by the yellow or orange summer flowers, more than the convenience of

breaking the leaf and applying directly to sores. With similar properties to Aloe Vera, it is indispensable in the battlefield of your back garden. (Excellent for sunburn, insect bites and rashes too.)

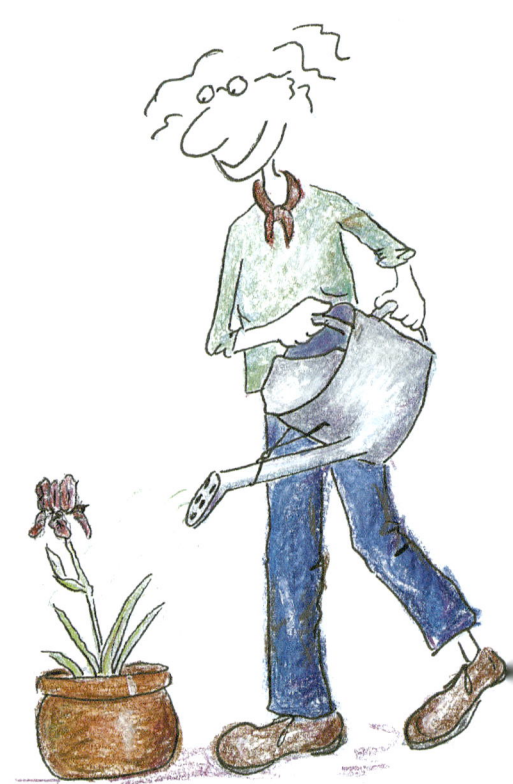

Lemon balm (Melissa officinalis) - children will enjoy the fresh lemon scent, pluck the leaves for their games, later to be calmed by its sedative qualities, sneaked into tea.

Berries - (if they'll let them get ripe), strawberries, raspberries, loganberries etc. Need I say more ...

Nasturtium - the lure of nasturtiums in their variety of warm colours is quite irresistible. Fortunately nature provides this herb in abundance, leaving some for colds and flu.

Creeping thyme - delicious for walking and lying on. As it flowers for a short period in spring there is a brief season of bees to contend with.

Honeysuckle - all form of honeysuckle will delight the largest form of nectar foraging species.

Dill and Fennel - their anise or licorice taste make them popular herbs to chew in the garden. In fact the seeds from each of these plants were given by the American pilgrims to their children to allay hunger during long church sermons, becoming know as 'Meeting House Seed'.

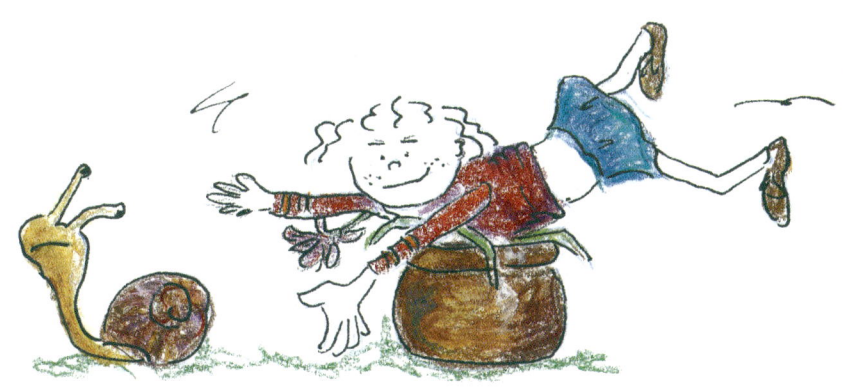

Catnip - a wonderful plant to grow for children. The two main varieties are Catnip, Nepeta mussinii and catmint Nepeta cataria. Which one is mint and which one is nip, varies according to interpretation; these are generally considered correct. Both plants lure kitties to them by imitating the odour of cat pheromones. One need not explain the resultant amourous behaviour of kitties towards the plant to your five year old.

BUTTERFLIES

Luring 'butterfliwes' into the garden enchants every child. Some species of children will need to be persuaded that butterflies benefit greatly if allowed to remain attached to their wings, particulary when still alive. Others will need reminding that a giddy pollinator is more endearing than one with a pin inserted through its middle. (Longevity is not a scorecard in butterflies' lives, so naturally deceased members can be found!)

Many herbs will serve the purpose of butterfly farming and should be planted in and around children's gardens or play areas. In general purple and blue flowers (e.g. lavender) do the best enticing. Other species to plant are golden rod, valerian, honeysuckle, hyssop, origanum sp, viola, lemon balm, sage, wild garlic and chives.

HERBS FOR AILING WILD THINGS

Children, who enjoy playing 'Lord of the Flies' in your garden, can often be interrupted by sores, cuts, bruises etc. Herbs are brilliant for cleansing and healing, as well as for when illness interrupts play. Many are febrifuges or diaphoretic and will thus lower a fever by encouraging perspiration. Other herbs will fight infection or help develop a strong immune system, particularly as herbal remedies support, rather than suppress immunity. Herbs will also sustain and strengthen the body.

You may find difficulty in persuading children to down the magic potion. Some will drink tea with honey; others will take a tincture in water. Fruit juice can also be used to hide herbal remedies in. Creams can be made or bought.

The following herbs are useful to have in your garden and home for children's ailments:

Lemon Balm - *insomnia, anti-oxidants to reduce inflammation - burns, cuts etc*

Catmint - *flu, colic, colds, reduce fever, measles, get restless child to sleep, flatulence, diarrhoea, upset tummies*

Fennel - *indigestion, colic, carminative, they love chewing it*

Lavender - *insomnia, calming*

Calendula - *cuts and scrapes, nappy rash, infusion to reduce the swelling in mumps*

German Chamomile - *reduce fever*

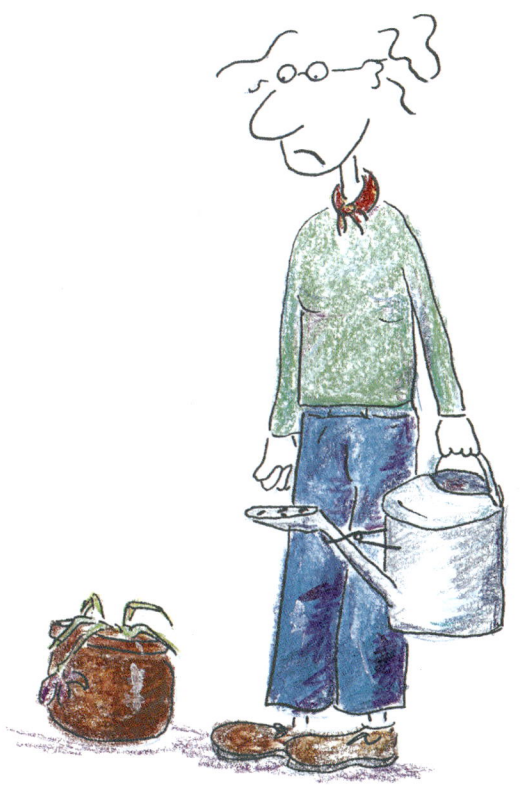

AILMENTS AND THEIR HERBAL TREATMENT:

nappy rash - *comfrey (in moderation) and calendula, both heal skin conditions.*

cuts and bruises - *yarrow staunches bleeding.*

calendula - *antiseptic.*

stings and burns - *bulbinella, houseleek, lavender (infusion or diluted oil).*

burns - *St. John's Wort oil, comfrey cream.*

colic - *dill, fennel, chamomile, ginger, peppermint. Infusions can be drunk by breastfeeding mothers; be aware that many stimulate milk flow and should be avoided if prone to mastitis. Bottle fed babies can have a teaspoon of infusion added to bottles. Infusions of these herbs can also be added to bath water – a quarter of a cup to a baby bath.*

earache - *echinacea internally, externally - mullein oil.*

ringworm - *calendula, garlic, tea tree.*

chicken pox rash - *elder flower or rosemary and calendula wash: 30g to 850ml boiling water. Cool, strain and apply to rash with cloth. Calendula tincture is also very useful, diluted and applied, helps with itching and healing of spots.*

measles rash - *tsp of distilled witch hazel with 250ml water, sponge on rash. Infusion of lavender is very soothing: tsp in cup of boiling water, cool and strain. Catnip infusion.*

teething - *syrup made from marshmallow root, reduces soreness in gums, add 3 tsps of syrup to baby's food or drink.*

ANGELICA'S SOUP RECIPE

you will need:
one beat up doll's cooking pot
one plastic spoon from your teaset
a garden
water

Fill your pot with water and a little white
sand from the sandpit, stir and slowly add
brown sand from the garden. When your
mixture has reached the consistency of
soup, walk around the garden picking
your favourite smelling herbs. Add and stir
occasionally. Recommended herbs: lavender, rosemary, nasturtium flowers, whole
chillis, catnip, sage, rose petals, scented
geranium leaves, lemon verbena and a
few blades of grass. A few empty snail
shells and ants will add to the flavour.
Serve at garden temperature.

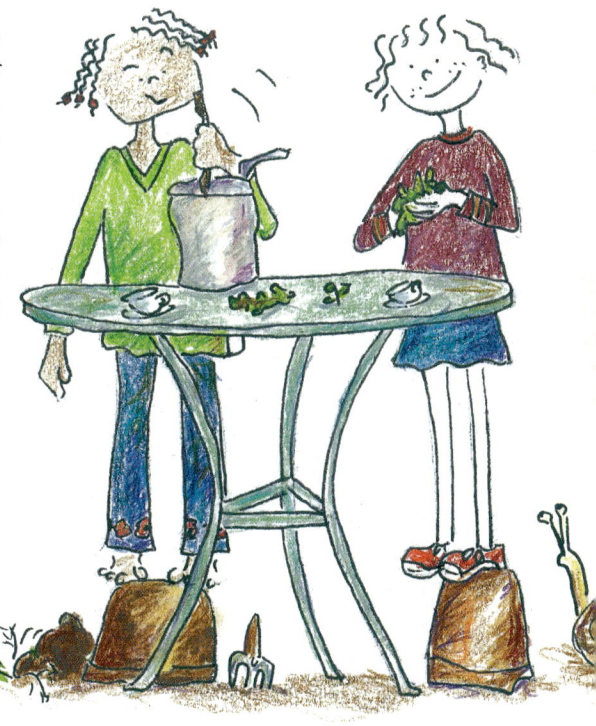

the sick bed

Such succulent skin,
for cacti to enter in,
leaves a prickled child,
without manners mild,
as operation tweezer extracts each botanical pin,

Thus Iris must find

a plant that is kind,

with orange blooms and edgy rind:

The aloe that grows in Angelica's garden of spikes,
Iris embraces and dissolves her dislikes,

with this antidote

of note,

which soothes and heals,

the pain Angelica feels.
Meanwhile as the salve is applied
word is spread wide

that at snailish pace,

the snails must race,

as Iris has detected,
how the munching snails have been protected,
and so the sense of emigration
slides through the mollusc nation.
The snails begin a mass exodus to Basil's garden,

enabling a mother to grant her daughter pardon.

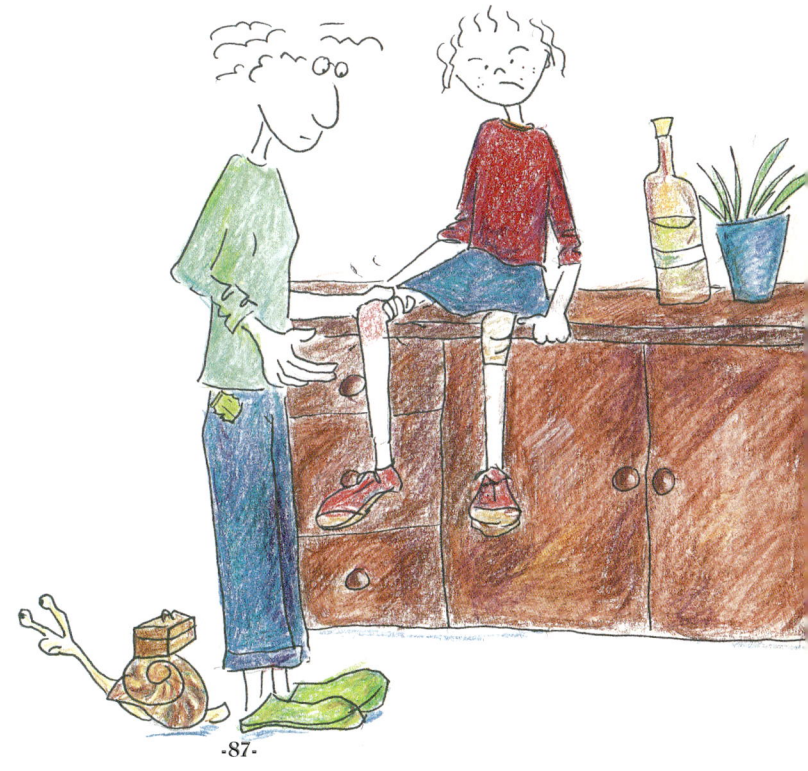

Many of us spent our childhoods nursing the imaginary ailments of our friends and siblings with medicines like dandelion leaves and mud. As an adult you will be delighted to know that you can continue this practice quite risk-free, by using many common, but safe herbal remedies. As long as you adhere to a reasonable dosage it will enable you to practice without having to scramble around for bail money. There is an endless inventory of herbs and the maladies they enjoy playing doctor-doctor on, but the common herbs, usually a pluck away from you, will astound you with their multiple uses.

Recommended herbs:
Thyme (Thymus vulgare)
antiseptic, anti-fungal, anti-bacterial, anti-catarrhal
Sage (Salvia officinalis)
both anti-bacterial and antiseptic, anti-cattarhal
Chamomile
antiseptic, anti-inflammatory, anti-fungal, anti-bacterial
Oregano (Oreganum vulgare)
both anti-bacterial and antiseptic
Elder (Sambucus nigra)
flowers - anti-catarrhal, leaves - expectorant
Nasturtium (Topaelum majus) *seed*
antibiotic, leaves - anti-bacterial
Hyssop (Hyssopus officinalis)
antiseptic and anti-viral, expectorant, anti-cattarhal
Garlic (Allium sativum)
anti-fungal, anti-viral and anti-bacterial, antiseptic, anti-catarrhal, expectorant

As like cures like, so we should seek out the dissatisfied plants in our time of grumpiness, caused by distended sinuses, sore throats and oozing noses. Whatever the cause, be sure to pursue the crabby species, like thyme, chamomile, sage, oregano and hyssop who, as you can see, are ANTI-everything. On the subject of dribbly noses, be it from hayfever or colds, elder comes highly recommended and will also deal a nasty blow to post-nasal drips. Another well-used and effective folk remedy for colds is garlic, which can be taken in capsule form or added raw to food. Stay in bed and you'll offend only the fleas and bed bugs by the odour you radiate.

Be sure to have a handful of nasturtium leaves and flowers nearby to fight the crusade against microbes. Leaves and flowers fight respiratory bacteria without destroying intestinal flora and the seed contains a natural antibiotic.

Use any or all of these as an infusion for any dissatisfied area from your chest up to your throat, mouth, nose and sinuses. Herbal infusions can also be inhaled in a steam bath in order to open congested sinuses or chests. Sore throats will benefit from a gargle of any of the above herbs.

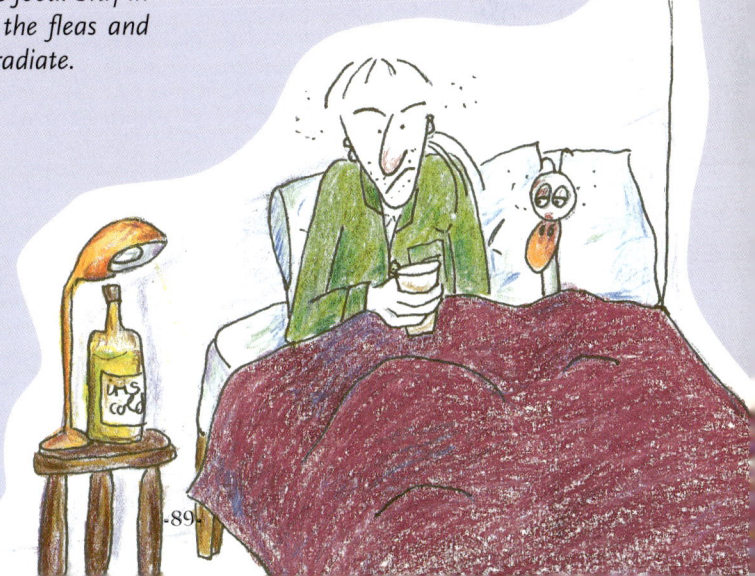

INSOMNIA AND STRESS

Recommended herbs:
Lavender (Lavendula sp.) - *sedative, carminative, anti-depressant, nervine*
Chamomile - *carminative, sedative, nervine*
Lemon Balm (Melissa officinalis) - *carminative, anti-depressant, aromatic*

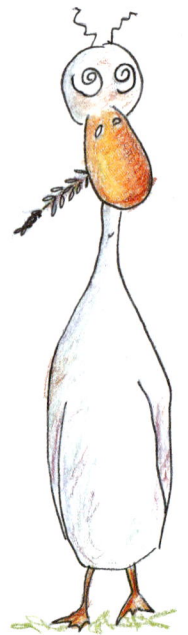

Lavender with its extended family boasts its own nepotistic United Nations, with species originating from the Mediterranean, India and Canary Islands! To add to the confusion it calls itself either French, Spanish or Italian and even has cultivars from England and Australia.

Regardless of its origins, lavender will soothe, calm and relax you; changing the internal presto forte metronome to a gentle lullaby, so much so that it will soothe mild insomnia. Chamomile will gently join lavender in the quest for calmness, especially if the subject of stress is a sleep-wary baby. *Add six drops of essential oil or 1/4 cup of an infusion of the above herbs to a bath to ease him/her into slumber.*

If your stress levels have slumped you into the dumps, then lemon balm and lavender should be combined for their anti-depressant qualities. Add a few drops of the essential oils (the essential oil of lemon balm is known as Melissa) to a bath to lift a crestfallen spirit.

ACHES AND PAINS

Recommended herbs:
Lavender - *anti-spasmodic, rubefacient*
Oregano (Oreganum vulgare) -
stimulant, rubefacient
Elder - *vulnerary, emollient*
Comfrey - *astringent*
Hyssop - *vulnerary, anti-spasmodic*

Make a bath of one or a combination of the herbs for aches and pains, be they of rheumatic origin or from coaxing your ligaments into a new yoga pose. Rub lavender or oregano into your temples to relieve headaches.

OW!

Recommended herbs:
Cuts, scrapes,bruises and burns
Lavender - *antiseptic*
Thyme - *anti-microbial, astringent, vulnerary*
Aloe Vera - *speeds cell regeneration*
Calendula - *anti-inflammatory, anti-microbial, analgesic*
Oregano (Vulgare) - *antiseptic*
Comfrey - *contains cell renewing allantoin*
St John's Wort (Hypericum perforatum)
- *flowering tops are anti-viral and astringent*

Caught unawares by the chopping knife, or victim to your children's collisions with the tarmac? Be certain to have some lavender essential oil ready for those painful faux pas. Add to this thyme, oregano and calendula, in cream or tincture form, as an invaluable antiseptic wound cleanser and healer.

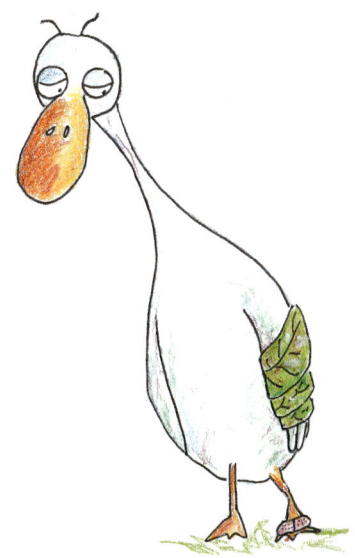

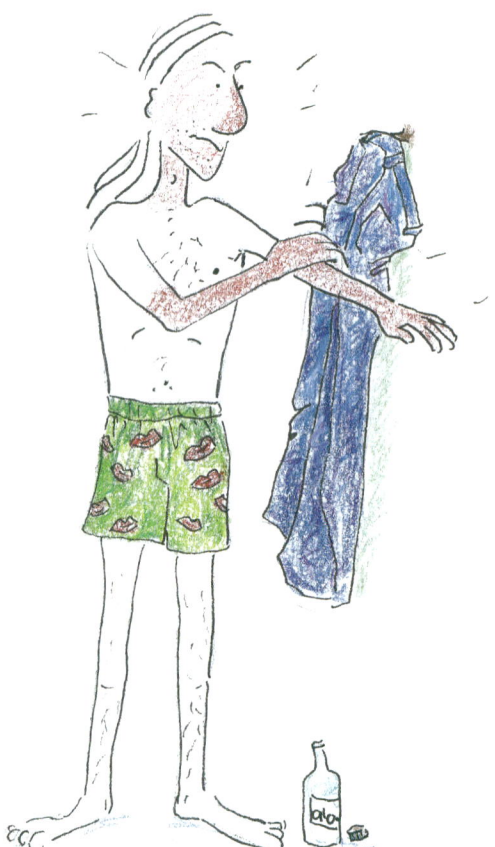

Post ozone hole discovery, fewer people walk around glowing with the pride of a roast sausage after a day stretched under the sun, but if you do become an unwitting victim of solar power, it is essential to remedy your sausage skin. Take a bath of lavender oil or smooth on soothing lotions of aloe or calendula. St John's Wort oil will also soothe and heal sunburn as it improves circulation to the area, thereby also making it useful for inflammation, wounds, bruises and varicose veins. This oil is made by macerating the flowers in oil, but can be bought at a chemist or health shop.

Comfrey is another essential wound herb, as it contains allantoin which hastens cell renewal in damaged muscles and broken bones. (It is not for nothing that it was known as knitbone.) Apply a comfrey leaf poultice to bruises, sprains and cuts. Home made or bought cream can also be applied to wounds, burns and arthritic joints.

INDIGESTION, STOMACHACHE

Recommended herbs:
Dill - *carminative, anti-spasmodic, anti-emetic*
Thyme - *carminative, anti-spasmodic, tonic*
Calendula - *tonic, cholagogue*
Chamomile Nobile - *anti-spasmodic, bitter, tonic*
Comfrey - *demulcent*
Hyssop - *anti-spasmodic, tonic*
Peppermint

Bellies have a way of behaving separately to the rest of us. You will find that your mouth is perfectly content to receive food your stomach will not. Other parts of your body are never indulgent enough to make your entire anatomy feel punished by your mouth's misdemeanour.

At other times stomachs are subject to very uncomfortable 'bugs' that produce momentary religious conversions at the pain. However, being essentially indispensable organs they do deserve some molly coddling. Whatever the cause of your discomfort, anti-spasmodic herbs will lessen the agony.

Dill, fennel, thyme and peppermint come highly recommended.

If you still wish to play culinary Russian roulette with your stomach, ensure that herbs like thyme, hyssop or sage accompany fatty foods, to aid digestion and hopefully prevent gastric punishment. If this fails follow your meal with an infusion of tummy herbs such as thyme, calendula, dill or peppermint, which are particularly good for indigestion.

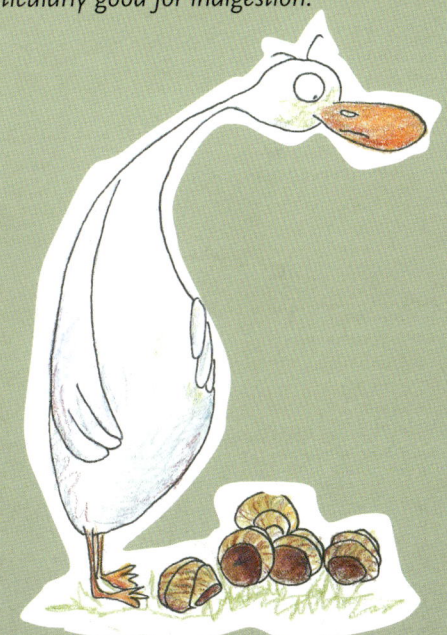

Parents of a colicky baby are often too familiar with dill water, eventually resorting to downing the bottle oneself to induce any kind of wind. This desperation can be of benefit to breastfeeding mothers, as dill also promotes breast milk. The rest of us can simply use dill for its anti-spasmodic activity when we are at the mercy of gastric disturbances.

More serious conditions such as gastric and duodenal ulcers will find calendula and comfrey soothing and healing on the intestinal mucosa.

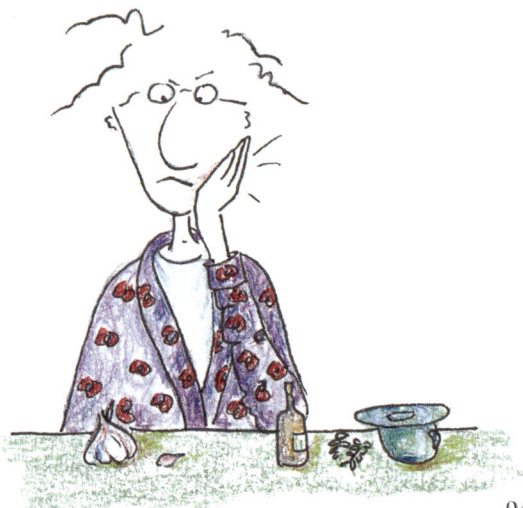

REMEDIES FROM THE TOOTH MOUSE

Recommended herbs:

Garlic	**Lemon Balm**
Yarrow	**Peppermint**
Tarragon	**Marjoram**

Toothache is, to say the least, rather unpleasant. Worst of all most toothache occurs at night or over a week-end, forcing you to endure hours of agony and sleeplessness or alternatively rather huge after-hours dental bills (causing further pain). There are many herbs said to ease toothache; I swear by none of these, having never tried any, but perhaps they will come to mind when your tooth is on holiday three days from civilisation and relaxes its guard against intruding bacteria. The following home remedies may just surface from your aching brain.

Garlic. Yes garlic. Pack a decaying tooth with garlic for pain relief. It is sure to get those bacteria marching back to civilisation and dental washes, but perhaps only to be used as a matter of emergency or prior to a visit to an insensitive dentist.

If you wish for a more sociable option, a lemon balm infusion is recommended, as well as a few drops of marjoram or peppermint oil on the tooth that is holding the rest of your mouth hostage.

Yarrow and tarragon leaves are also advised. I am sure most tarragon will shrivel at the thought of being a dental aid, but it is probably the most pleasant tasting! Don't forget to remove any offending green or smelly herbal material before you finally limp to the dentist.

MAKING HERBAL PREPARATIONS

The most desirable way of taking herbal potions is always fresh from the garden, but dried is an adequate substitute. Use one third the amount of dried herbs to the fresh herb dosage. The following methods of herbal usage are centuries old and worth their weight in gold.

INFUSIONS/TISANES

With an infusion soft parts of the herb are used, usually three tsp fresh herb (one tsp dried) to 600ml boiled water. The water is poured over the preferably bruised herb into a ceramic or glass vessel. This is then covered to prevent the evaporation of essential oils, then left to seep for five to 10 minutes. Infusions are best drunk as fresh as possible the same day as certain bacteria are not deterred by the infusion's healing qualities.

Standard dosage:
one cup three times a day

Catarrh and colds: borage, comfrey and hyssop
Feverish colds: elderflower, peppermint and yarrow
Constipation: basil, dandelion, licorice root, parsley, feverfew
Cuts: yarrow, comfrey, calendula
Depression: St John's Wort (strengthens and calms nerves)
Indigestion: peppermint
Earache: chamomile (warm): a few drops in the ear, to dissolve wax – a strong infusion of warm marjoram
Eyes: chamomile, hyssop
Flatulence: dill, peppermint, aniseed
Haemorrhoids: parsley leaf internally, apply witch hazel externally

Headaches: lemon balm, rosemary, sage, thyme, lavender, chamomile
Travel sickness: cold basil drunk before journey
Nausea: peppermint, lemon balm
Anxiety and tension: lavender, lemon balm, hyssop
Insomnia: chamomile, elder, bergamot, dill, anise, fennel
Sore throats: gargle with one or all: angelica, peppermint, lemon balm
Toothache: lemon balm
Hangover: thyme
Thrush: tea tree, garlic, calendula – use as douche
Blood cleansing: hyssop
Tonic: hyssop

Standard dosage: one cup three times a day
Coughs: comfrey root, marshmallow root, elecampane root, white horehound
Stye: hot comfrey root

● DECOCTION

Contrary to an infusion where the parts are never boiled, a decoction is a method used to break down harder plant parts such as bark, roots or seeds. These are bruised and then boiled in a covered pot. The general dosage is 25g to one litre cold water, slowly bringing to boil and then simmering gently until the liquid has reduced by half. Strain, cool and use.

HERBAL BATHS

Herbal baths can be used medicinally rather than merely for pleasure, as the skin will carry the active ingredients through the blood to body organs. In the same manner foot and hand baths can be undertaken instead of taking an oral remedy. This can be useful for children who develop lock-jaw at the sight of your potions.

Herbal baths can be taken with a few drops of essential oils, a few millimetres of herbal bath oil, or a quick and easy way is to wrap some herbs in a bag (a non-smelly cotton sock will do) and run under the tap. Alternatively make an infusion and add to bathwater.

COMPRESSES

Compresses appear to be old fashioned methods of healing but are well worth resuscitating. Usually they are cold, but a hot compress is best when one is trying to draw an alien substance out of the body. To make a compress, a piece of folded cloth is dipped into a cold infusion and laid on the skin. When the cloth has been warmed by the body it should be removed and the process repeated three or four times.

Hot: *Acne, pimples, boils – elder, thyme, sorrel*

Cold: *Bruises, sprains – witch-hazel, calendula*

Eye: *inflamed eyelids – eyebright, fennel, calendula*

Sunburn: *witch hazel, angelica, salad burnett, elderflowers*

POULTICE

A poultice is used to soothe as well as draw out poisons. They can also be used on cuts and sores. Soft herbs are chosen and wrapped in a cloth. The middle is then immersed in boiled water until the herbs are soft. Take the ends and squeeze out the excess water before applying to the affected area. Place on the skin immediately and repeat when the cloth has cooled. This can be repeated at least three times before the herbs loose effect.

Acne, pimples, boils: *hops, marshmallow leaves or roots, thyme leaves or flowers*

Bruises, sprains: *comfrey, hyssop, hypericum, catnip, peppermint pelargonium*

Stye: *pounded seeds of nasturtium*

Headache: *crushed peppermint leaves on forehead*

Wounds: *hyssop*

OINTMENTS

Making ointments allows us to imagine ourselves as witches, just omitting the eye of frog part. Finding the right base for ointments can be complicated. Most books recommend lard or petroleum jelly. Lard can be a tad tricky for vegetarians, and petroleum jelly is a by-product of the petro-chemical industry, which does not quite make it free of toxins. Lanolin is another possibility although some people are allergic to it. Beeswax is a relatively problem free solution.

The following recipes work on the same basis of melting the substrate in a pot followed by the herbs.

Lard: *225g of lard in pan, when melted add 25g of crushed herbs. Simmer 30 minutes*
Petroleum jelly and lanolin: *25g crushed herb to 112g base. Simmer 20 minutes*

Beeswax: *add 125ml olive oil to 25g beeswax, and 25g herb. Simmer 20 minutes.*
With all methods strain through a cloth into a sterilised jar. They are best kept in the fridge for a longer life.
And remember a little witches' spell might just improve the quality.

Cuts and abrasions: *lady's mantle, comfrey, hypericum, calendula*
Sunburn: *calendula, elderflower*

TINCTURE

Infusion and the like do not have much of a shelf life, which brings us to tinctures. These are great to make as it enables you to feel at one with Hippocrates and the boys, and at the same time create really effective herbal remedies. Best of all they have a shelf life of approximately two years, sometimes longer. Those who wish to avoid the alcohol can use apple cider vinegar instead, using the same method.

Pure alcohol is required, preferably vodka or cane (save the whiskey for the hot toddy), but stay away from the deathly laboratory alcohol. The general dosage is 45g crushed or powdered herb to 600ml alcohol in an airtight jar. This must be left in a warm place for two to three weeks and shaken daily. You will see that it is ready when the alcohol becomes greenish and the herbs anaemic looking. This should then be strained into brown bottles, as light will weaken their shelf life.

Tinctures are generally taken three times a day, 15 drops in a glass of water.

WHEN NOT TO TAKE

Do not take any concoctions or potions when pregnant or breastfeeding without consulting your medical practitioner. Seemingly harmless herbs can do damage where least expected. Not all herbs are appropriate for babies; be certain that they can be used, especially essential oils. Some seemingly innocuous plants are poisonous or only some parts of well used plants are. Be certain before you dose; keep the bail money on the monopoly board.

GROWING TIPS

Alfalfa/Lucerne (Medigo sativa)
60-90cm, full sun
rich soil
self sows readily
can be invasive in some areas
roots high in nitrogen content
dig in to enrich soil
use young leaves

Aloe sp.
Cape Aloe (Aloe ferox) 2-4m
Aloe Vera 30-40cm, full sun
very well-drained, coarse, sandy soil
frost sensitive
slow growing, but worth it

Angelica (Angelica archangelica)
60cm biannual, semi-shade
moist, rich soil, slightly acid
sow seeds as soon as possible as they
cannot be stored
will self sow easily
cut off flower head to prolong life to
three or four years

Artichoke (Cynara scolymus)
1.5cm, full sun, protect from wind
well-drained rich soil
prone to aphids in wet winters,
but generally survive this

Basil (Ocimum basilicum)
30-50 cm, annual, full sun
(avoid harsh midday sun and wind)
well-drained soil
important to dead head flowers to
prolong life of plant
many varieties suitable for containers
sow seeds only when very hot weather

Bay (Laurus nobilis)
6-10m, full sun/semi-shade
rich well-drained soil
protect from wind and frost
very slow growing
suitable for container

Bergamot (Monarda didyma)
60cm, full sun/semi-shade
rich, light soil, will benefit from addition
of bonemeal
lift and divide every 3-4 years
suitable for large container
flowers from mid-summer

Borage (Borago officinalis)
starflower/herb of joy
32cm, annual, full sun
average to rich soil
self sows readily
plant in clumps to support each other

Bulbinella (Bulbine frutescens)
30cm, full sun
well-drained average soil
will grow well in hot places
very drought resistant
lift and divide when overcrowded
suitable for container

Calendula (Calendula officinalis)
30-50cm, annual, full sun
sow in spring and summer in northern
hemisphere and autumn or spring   in
southern hemisphere
well-drained, slightly acid, sandy soil
self sows readily, but seedlings prone to
caterpillars

Catnip (Nepeta cataria) creeping
Catmint (Nepeta mussinii)
40cm, full sun
well-drained soil
cut back after flowering
protect from kitties until it has reached
a size able to take them on

Cayenne (Capsicum frutescens)
60cm, full sun
rich soil
will get through winter in warm climates,
but protect from cold winds, otherwise
treat as annual or try moving it to sunny
position indoors
cut back after fruiting

Chamomile, Roman (Chamaemelum nobile)
10-30cm, German (Matricaria recutita)
50cm, full sun/ semi-shade
well-drained sandy soil, slightly acid
flower in summer
C. nobile can be grown in lawn
fresh apple-y scent.
M. recutita self sows readily

Chaste Tree (Vitex agnes castus)
6m deciduous, full sun
well-drained acid soil
protect from wind

Chervil (Anthriscus cerefolium)
30-50cm annual, semi-shade
well-drained, light, rich soil
sow in situ

Chicory (Cichorium intybus)

30-50cm, full sun to shade
good, alkaline soil
dip up roots in autumn, remove leaves
and replant in sandy soil
the new leaves will be white and less bitter

Chives (Allium schoenoprasum)

20cm, full sun/semi-shade
most soils, but enjoys well composted
suitable for container
lift and divide every 3-4 years
purple flowers in summer

Garlic Chives (Allium tuberosum)

40cm, full sun/semi-shade
most soils, but enjoys well composted
suitable for container
lift and divide every 3-4 years
white flowers in summer

Comfrey (Symphytum officinale)

1m, full sun/semi-shade
most soils
use as soil conditioner in bad soils
will die back in winter in some climates
easily propagated from root cuttings
**do not take internally unless under
supervision of a health practitioner**

Coriander (Coriandrum sativum)

20-30cm, annual, full sun/ semi-shade
(in harsh conditions)
best in rich moist soil
first leaves are used in curries etc, they
then become more feathery and less
pallateable, leave to go to seed and use,
or sow.

Dandelion (Taraxacum officinale)

10-20cm, full sun
self sows readily (as most gardeners
will testify)
grows in most soils, but best in
well-composted soil
water well in hot weather
best grown in container so that it
can be controlled

Dill (Anethum graveolens)

60cm, full sun/semi-shade
well-drained soil, slightly acid
sow in situ all year round (except winter)

Echinacea (Echinacea purpurea)

60- 120cm, full sun
deciduous rhizome
well-composted and well-drained soil
flowers in summer

Elder (Sambucus nigra)
6-10m, full sun/semi-shade
will only bear berries in climates where
temperature reaches below freezing

Fennel (Foeniculum vulgare)
1-3m, full sun/semi-shade
grows in most soil, but best in richer soil
flowers in summer

Garlic (Allium sativum)
60cm, full sun
well-drained, alkaline soil, well-composted
plant cloves 5 cm deep
plant in autumn, to harvest in spring

Rose Scented Geranium (Pelargonium graveolens 60cm-1m and P. capitatum
30-60cm)
full sun/semi-shade
well-drained soil
can be grown indoors in cold climates

Ginger (Zingiber officinale)
1m, full sun
light, moist soil
can be propagated from cuttings of
shooting rhizome
grows well in tropical, sub-tropical
climates
lift rhizomes 6-12 months after planting
use fresh or dried

Honeysuckle (Lonicera sp.)
4-10m, depending on species, full sun
well-drained, well-composted soil ideal
with roots in shade and foliage in sun
hardy plants, grows well anywhere

Cape Honeysuckle (Teocomaria capensis)
2m, full sun, semi-shade
any soil, add compost
popular as hedge

Horseradish (Armoricia rusticana)
1m, full sun
well-drained. well-composted soil
propagate from root cuttings in spring
plant at 5cm deep, 30cm apart
roots only ready after two to three years,
dig up in autumn and store in sand in
cold, dark place for winter, or grate and
pickle

Houseleek (Sempervivum tectorum)
10cm, full sun
well-drained and thin gritty sand -
prefer very little soil
flowers after many years and then dies,
but will have produced enough offsets
by then

Hyssop (Hyssopus officinalis)
45cm, full sun
light, well-drained soil
cut back after flowering

Lamb's Ear (Stachys lanata)
spreading, low growing
full sun/semi-shade
pale lilac flowers in summer
well-drained soil, water well

Lavender (Lavendula sp.)
heights vary according to species
full sun
well-drained soil, slightly alkaline
cut back after flowering

Lemon Balm (Melissa officinalis)
40cm, sun/semi-shade
moist, rich soil
often dies back in winter
cut back after flowering
prone to frost

Lemon Grass (Cymbopogon citrates)
1-1.5m, full sun
well-drained, well-composted soil

Lemon Verbena (Aloysia triphylla)
60- 130cm, full sun
frost sensitive
average alkaline soil
deciduous
will do well in large container

Licorice (Glycyrrhiza glabra)
1m, full sun
deep, rich, sandy soil
to produce good quality roots, prevent
from flowering
prone to frost

Lovage (Levisticum officinale)
1-2m, semi-shade
well-drained, rich, moist soil
lasts about four years
dies back in winter
prone to frost - protect with thick mulch

Common Marjoram/Oregano
(Origanum vulgare) 90cm

Pot Marjoram
Origanum onites low growing

Sweet Marjoram (Origanum marjorana)
30-60cm, full sun
well-drained soil
cut back after flowering
spreading varieties do not do well
in containers

Marigold (Tagetes sp.)
annual, full sun
average soil
sow seeds in spring, nip out centres
to encourage bushing

Marshmallow (Althaea officinalis)
90cm, full sun
damp rich soil
dies back in winter
attractive light pink flowers in summer

Mint (Mentha sp.)
Peppermint (Mentha x piperita)
all mints can be very invasive
require a moist rich soil, and are heavy
feeders
mint can be grown in containers but are
happy where they can roam free
replace soil annually
compost regularly for a lush supply
cut back after flowering
some mints die back in winter

Nasturtium (Tropaelum majus)
30-50cm, annual, full sun/semi-shade
grows in most soils (rich soil will encourage leaf rather than flower growth)
self-sow readily

Parsley Curly (Petroselinum crispum)
20cm

Parsley Flat or Italian (Petroselinum crispum var. neopolitanum)
20-30cm, full sun/semi-shade
rich, moist soil
parsley does not like having its roots
tampered with when transplanting
flat-leaved variety is hardiest and grows
best
both varieties will benefit from
addition of well-diluted chicken manure

Pennyroyal (Mentha pulegium)
creeping
semi-shade/shade
moist, rich soil
cut back after flowering

Pennywort *(Centella asiatica)*
creeping
full sun/semi-shade
most soils, but will do well in
moist rich soil
propagate from runners which send
out roots

Ribwort *(Plantago lanceolata)*
25cm, full sun
average soil
grows as weed in some places

Rocket *(Eruca vesicaria ssp. sativa)*
50cm, full sun
well-composted soil
self sows readily
best grown in clumps to support each
other
tendency to bolt in hot climates (best
sown in autumn)

Rosemary *(Rosmarinus officinalis)*
1m, full sun
well-drained soil, slightly alkaline soil, will
benefit from addition of bonemeal
can live up to 30 years
many varieties with flowers varying in
shades of blue, as well as pink and white
varieties

Rue *(Ruta graveolens)*
60cm, full sun
well-drained average soil
cut back after flowering
**rue is poisonous to livestock - take care
where you plant it, it also can also cause
allergic reactions from handling it!**

Sage *(Salvia officinalis)*
30cm, full sun
well-drained soil essential especially in wet
areas
sage can be a complete mystery, dying for
no reasonable explanation. It is a matter
of giving it sufficient water as it will not
recover from drought, but at the same
time it doesn't like to get its feet wet!
cut back after flowering

Salad Burnett *(Sanguisorba minor)*
20cm, full sun
average soil
clusters of tiny red flowers in summer

Santolina/Cotton Lavender *(Santolina chamaecyparissus, S. neopolitana)*
50-80cm
well-drained, slightly alkaline soil
yellow button flowers in summer
cut back to keep from getting straggly

Selfheal (Prunella vulgaris) ground cover
sun/semi-shade
most soils
attractive pink/purple flowers
can be grown in a lawn

Senna (Senna alexandrina)
full sun
well-drained, average soil, add compost
sow pods or keep for use
unattractive in winter, but recovers in summer

Stinging Nettle (Urtica urens)
annual 30cm (Urtica dioca)
perennial 1.5m full sun
moist rich soil
use only new leaves
does not do well in container -
heavy feeder

St John's Wort (Hypericum perforatum)
30-90cm full sun/semi-shade
average soil
requires a lot of water in summer

Southernwood (Artemesia abrotanum)
60cm full sun/semi-shade
well-drained soil
prune regularly to keep shape

Tansy (Tanecetum vulgare)
50cm-1m, full sun/semi-shade
average slightly alkaline soil
propagate by root division
grows in clumps
yellow button-like flowers
may die back in winter

Tarragon (Artemesia dracunculus)
60cm, full sun
rich, well-drained soil
dies back in winter

Thyme (Thymus vulgare)
30cm, full sun
well-drained soil, roots do not like wet conditions
cut back after flowering
many varieties of thyme, most edible, many creeping - when in flower attractive mass of tiny white to pink to magenta flowers

Vietnamese Coriander (Rau rau)
(Polygonum odoratum)
30cm, full sun to semi-shade in very dry climates
tender perennial, winter indoors in cold climates
rich, moist soil
water well

Watercress (Nasturtium officinale)

low growing
full sun/semi-shade
grows well in water
grow in sunken container in pond (water
must be kept very fresh) or very damp
corner of the garden

Witchhazel (Hamamelis virginiana)

3-5m deciduous
sun or dappled shade
rich, acid soil

Wormwood (Artemesia absinthium)

50cm-1m, full sun
protect from wind
most soils
tiny yellow flowers in summer

Yarrow (Achillea millefolium)

30-60cm, full sun
well-drained, light soil
divide clumps 2-3 years

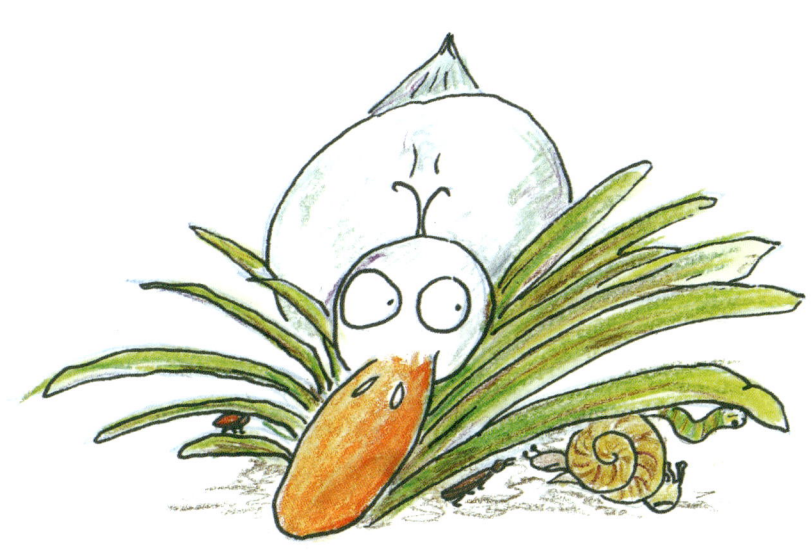

glossary

anti-catarrhal -
helps in battle against snot

anti-emetic -
helps with nausea and hopefully assists in keeping your dinner inside your stomach

anti-inflammatory -
substance which calms inflamed tissue

anti-microbial -
a crusader against invading germs and other baddies

anti-spasmodic -
calms down stomachs that are cramping or in spasm

aromatic -
substance that smells good, but also stimulates the digestive system. These are often added to less aromatic and tasty medicines to fool you into administering them

bitters -
a dreadful tasting substance that shocks your digestive system into working more effectively

astringent -
a substance that causes tissues to contract through binding of proteins, thereby assisting in wound healing

carminative -
a substance which is rich in volatile oils, both relaxing and stimulating the digestive system, helping with digestion and making one a tad less gaseous

catarrh -
excessive excretion of phlegm from the air passage

cholagogue -
good for gall bladder stimulation which is our bodies' very own laxative. Also useful for unwell gall bladders

colic -
abdominal pain and discomfort from intestinal wind

conjunctivitis -
infection of the mucous membrane of the eye

deciduous -
sheds its leaves in winter

demulcent -
soothes and heals inflamed internal body tissues

emollient -
soothes and heals inflamed external body tissue

enfleurage -
fat used to absorb plant's perfume for production of essential oil, used with fragile petals

expectorant -
a substance which helps lungs to cough up stubborn phlegm

febrifuge -
a substance which reduces fevers

mastitis -
inflammation of the breast in breastfeeding mothers

nervine -
tones and strengthens nervous system as well as stimulates or relaxes

rubefacient -
a substance which causes irritation when applied to skin; this calls blood from within to the surface, helping to alleviate internal pains

sedative -
a substance which alleviates stress by calming the nervous system, especially useful for 'frayed nerves' caused by stress

stimulant -
a substance that induces a wake up call for your entire body

tonic -
a substance that strengthens and enlivens body organs

vulnerary -
applied to cuts and wounds to assist healing

SOIL

sandy soil -
runs through your fingers when holding it

loamy soil -
stays in your hand, but pieces do not compact under pressure

clay -
forms a soft putty-like ball when squeezed

pH -
most plants will thrive in a soil with an neutral pH of 7, but those preferring acid soils require a pH below 7, whereas alkaline soils are above this margin.

Generally clay, coarse loam and peat soils are more acidic whereas loamy and chalky soils are more alkaline. This is not always the case though, thus to test your soil a pH kit can be bought from nurseries. Soils which have a reading too far on either end of the scale will not release nutrients and will require assistance.

Lime can be added to increase alkalinity, where acid soils are formed by the addition of sulphur. More convenient is a mulch of pine needles or well-rotted manure. Do not add lime and compost/manure at the same time. Regular addition of organic compost should ensure that your soil slowly builds up all the required minerals.

index

B

C

D

E

earache, 84, 95
earl grey tea, 69
earthworms, 73
eau de logne mint, 60
echinacea, 84
eczema, 72
elder, 88, 95, 96, 97, 98
elecampane, 96
eggs, 42
egyptians, 34
essential oils, 57, 59, 97
ethylene gas, 17
eyebright, 97
eyes, 95, 97

F

fennel, 17, 50 (insect bites), 34, 60,
       69, 81, 83, 96, 97
fever, 95
feverfew, 95
fishmoths, 51
flatulence, 23, 33, 34, 69, 70, 95
flu, 81
free radicals, 72
fungi, 75

G

gamma lineolic acid, 24
garlic, 15, 43 (anti-snail recipe), 89, 95,
       96
gastric ulcers, 23
geranium (rose), 60, 61, 70
ginger, 68
goldenrod, 82
gout, 23
green tea, 66

H

haemoglobin, 32, 33 (haemorrhoids),
       95 (hangover), 96
hayfever, 89
headaches, 67, 71, 95, 96, 97
heart, 59, 71
honeysuckle, 81
hormones, 25-26
horseradish, 26
houseleek, 50 (insect bites)
hypericum - see St. John's Wort
hyssop, 37, 60, 88, 89, 90, 93, 95, 96

I

infusion, 66, 72, 95, 96, 97
insect bites, 80
insomnia, 68, 71, 90, 96
immune system, 82
irritable bowels, 27

J

jasmine, 37
jojoba oil, 59
juniper, 60

K

kidneys, 70

L

lacewings, 48
ladybirds, 48
lady's mantle, 98
landcress, 35
lanolin, 98
lavender, 17, 51 (fish moths), 79
    (lavender and rosemary
    biscuits), 50 (insect bites), 60,
    79, 83, 84, 90, 91, 96
lamb's ear, 79
lard, 98

M

lemon balm, 50 (insect bites), 60, 71,
    81, 83, 90, 95, 96
lemongrass, 46 (anti-mosquito), 71
lemon verbena, 70
licorice, 69, 95
linseed oil, 48
liver, 22, 69
lovage, 32

marigold (tagetes), 15
marjoram, 14, 60, 62
marshmallow, 84, 96, 97
mealy bug, 48
measles, 84, 95
melissa, 90
menopause, 24
menstrual problems, 27
minerals, 24, 25, 27, 34, 72, 73, 75
mint, 15, 17, 23 (fish moths), 67, 80
molasses, 45 (pest control)
mosquitoes, 46 (control of)
mullein, 84

N

nappy rash, 72, 84, 89
nasturtium, 32, 37, 81
nausea, 38, 69, 70
nematodes, 15
nettle - see stinging nettle

O

oak, 75
oats, 50 (insect bites)
ointments, 98
olfactory, 56
oleum, 48
olive oil, 59
onion, 50(insect bites)
oregano, 62, 88, 89, 91

P

pain, 91
parsley, 31, 62, 95
pelargoniums, 70, 80, 97
pennyroyal, 46 (anti-mosquito), 47
        (anti-ant), 67
peppermint, 14, 15, 60, 93, 95, 97
petroleum jelly, 98
pests, 48, 73
post-nasal drip, 89
poultice, 97

pregnancy, 23, 24, 99
preservative, 61
pyrethurm, 50

R

rash, 50, 80
rheumatism, 23
ribwort, 50 (insect bites)
ringworm, 84
rocket, 32
rooibos, 72
rosemary, 50 (insect bites), 60, 61, 79,
        79 (rosemary and lavender
        biscuits), 96
roses, 15
rue, 17

S

sage, 14, 88, 89, 96
salad burnett, 32, 97
scale, 48
sedative, 70, 71, 81, 90
self heal, 49 (insect bites)
senna, 26
sinus, 89
skin, 92
slugs, 42-44, 30-39,
snails, 42-44 (snail traps)
sores, 80

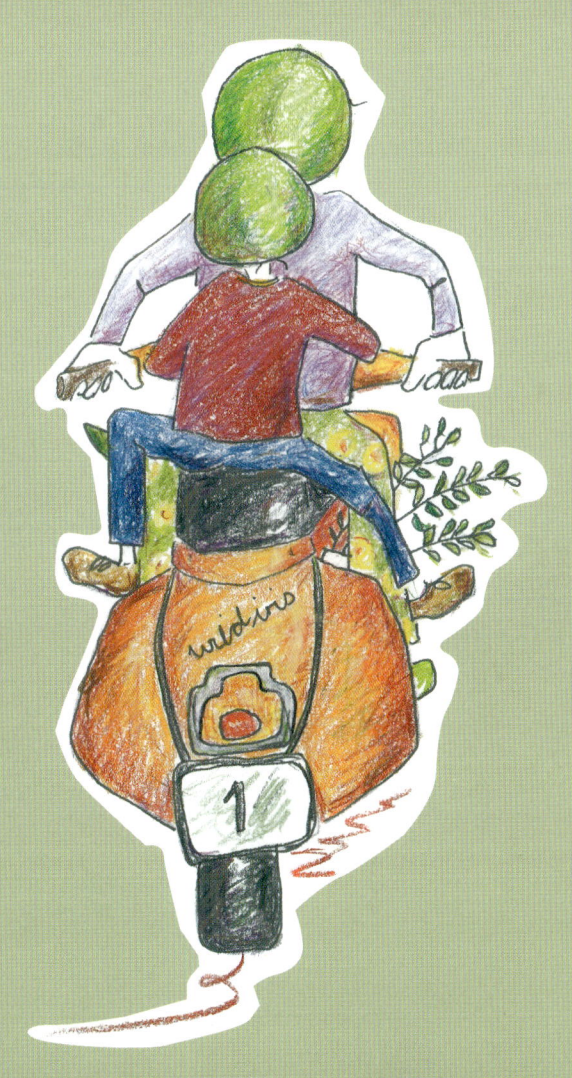

BIBLIOGRAPHY

-Boxer, Arabella; Back, Philippa, *The Herb Book,* Octopus Books Ltd, 1980

-Bremness, L, *Herbs, Eyewitness Handbooks,* Dorling Kindersley, 1994

-Garden Way Publishing, The Editors, *The Big Book of Gardening Skills, A Garden Way* Publishing Book, 1994

-Hey, Barbara, *The Illustrated Book of Herbs,* New Holland, 1996

-Hoffmann, David, *Holistic Herbal,* Element Boks Ltd, 1996

-McVicar, Jekka, *Jekka's Complete Herb Book,* Kyle Cathie Ltd, 1997

-Palmer, Eve, *The South African Herbal,* Tafelberg Publishers Ltd, 1985

-Reichardt, Irmela, *Natural Gardening,* Delta Books, 1993

-Roberts, Margaret, *Indigenous Healing Plants,* Southern Book Publishers, 1990

-Roberts, Margaret, *A-Z of Herbs,* Southern Book Publishers, 1993

- Van Wyk, Yvette, *First Aid With Herbs,* Blackwood Herbs, 1998

-Watkins, *Companion Plants,* London & Dulverton, 1967